Treating Articulation and Phonological Disorders in Children

Treating Articulation and Phonological Disorders in Children

Dennis M. Ruscello, PhD

Professor
Department of Speech Pathology and Audiology
College of Human Resources and Education
West Virginia University
Morgantown, West Virginia

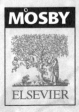

MOSBY

ELSEVIER

11830 Westline Industrial Drive
St. Louis, Missouri 63146

TREATING ARTICULATION AND PHONOLOGICAL
DISORDERS IN CHILDREN

ISBN: 978-0-323-03387-9

Notice

Neither the Publisher nor the Author assumes any responsibility for any loss or injury and/or damage to persons or property arising out of or related to any use of the material contained in this book. It is the responsibility of the treating practitioner, relying on independent expertise and knowledge of the patient, to determine the best treatment and method of application for the patient.

The Publisher

Library of Congress Control Number 2007931994

Vice President and Publisher: Linda Duncan
Acquisitions Editor: Kathy Falk
Managing Editor: Kristin Hebberd
Publishing Services Manager: Patricia Tannian
Project Manager: Jonathan M. Taylor
Design Direction: Mark Oberkrom
Chapter-opening photographs from Paul R: Language disorders from infancy through adolescence: assessment intervention, ed 3, St Louis, 2007, Mosby.

Printed in the United States of America

Last digit is the print number: 9 8 7 6 5 4 3 2 1

Working together to grow
libraries in developing countries

www.elsevier.com | www.bookaid.org | www.sabre.org

ELSEVIER   BOOK AID International   Sabre Foundation

This book is dedicated to
my colleagues at West Virginia University
and those researchers and practitioners
who have taught me so much during my 35 years of practice.

It is also dedicated to
the children with sound system disorders and their caregivers,
whom I have served and continue to serve and learn from each day.

Preface

There are large numbers of children with sound system disorders,* and these children are seen for assessment and treatment services by speech-language pathologists. Estimates suggest that approximately 80% of children with sound system disorders require clinical services. The etiology of sound system disorders is unknown for most children, but there are subgroups of children who have sound system disorders that are a function of structural, sensory, or neurological disorders. Our knowledge base in this area of communicative disorders has increased dramatically over the past 25 years because of developments in the professions of linguistics, cognitive psychology, and motor-skill learning, to name a few. In addition, researchers in our profession have systematically examined a number of different treatments and have developed an evidence base to support the treatments, which are based on dissimilar theoretical perspectives.

AUDIENCE AND NEED

The impetus for this book is the fact that the population of children with sound system disorders is heterogeneous. The heterogeneity requires that students in speech-language pathology and audiology programs, as well as practitioners of speech-language pathology, be aware of the different treatments so they may select the appropriate one. That is, treatment selection is a decision-making process that is a function of the clinician's education and clinical experience. It is not an arbitrary process based on the comfort level of the clinician with a particular sound

---

* The term *sound system disorders* refers to clinically significant sound production errors, which may have a phonetic or phonemic basis. The term *sound system disorders* will be used throughout this text in discussions of specific treatments for children who may exhibit phonetic (articulatory) and/or phonemic (phonological) production errors.

system treatment. The provider of services—whether that individual is a student under clinical supervision or a practitioner in the field—must carefully examine a child's sound system disorder and implement the appropriate treatment. In the case of a student clinician, the decision will be made in consultation with the clinical supervisor. This book contains a breadth of information that can be used to identify and implement the most appropriate treatment for a specific child.

UNIQUE CONTENT AND CONCEPTUAL APPROACH

An additional consideration in writing the book is that most current books address sound system disorders primarily from an unknown etiological perspective. This makes sense because most children with sound system disorders do not exhibit some identifiable etiology. However, it compels clinicians to identify other literature sources for low-incidence subgroups exhibiting different structural, sensory, or neurological causal factors. Generally, texts and other sources deal exclusively with a specific subgroup. For instance, a child born with a cleft of the lip and palate may demonstrate sound system errors that require special consideration when planning and implementing a treatment. It would be necessary to obtain a relevant text or literature source because most students and practitioners see such clients on an infrequent basis. This text contains specialized treatment information for the low-incidence subgroups in addition to individuals who have sound system disorders of unknown etiology. That is, this text is a compendium of different treatments that are employed for the population of children with sound system disorders.

ORGANIZATION

The first chapter is an introduction and presents the basic principles of the text. It discusses the heterogeneous nature of sound system disorders, discusses general programmatic issues, and introduces a treatment model that incorporates clinician, client, and caregiver variables. Information is presented regarding theories of learning and treatment factors that are important in planning, conducting, and evaluating treatment programs. Chapter 2 is an in-depth description of treatments that are currently used in the remediation of clients with sound system disorders of unknown etiology. The chapter is organized along the dichotomy of a motor learning approach (phonetic, traditional) versus a linguistic approach (phonemic, cognitive-linguistic); however, some treatments embody the features of both and are also included. Chapter 3 addresses treatment concepts for the motor speech disorders of childhood apraxia of speech (CAS) and dysarthria. Childhood apraxia of speech is conceptualized in the text as a deficit in planning and programming of skilled movement, whereas dysarthria is defined as an execution problem with articulatory movement.

Some clients with sound system disorders have coexisting anomalies of the oral speech mechanism. These structural differences can be minor problems, such as missing teeth, or major problems, such as cleft palate. Chapter 4 presents specific intervention protocols for these different structural problems, whereas Chapter 5 deals with the treatment of sound system disorders for children with hearing impairment. Hearing impairment is a variable that affects speech production, and certain treatment variables are important in developing a remediation plan. Chapter 6 addresses children who exhibit residual errors. Generally, children in this diagnostic category have not responded to traditional treatments, or they have maintained the sound system error after the expected period of developmental maturation. These children are limited in number and often need specialized treatments, such as the use of biofeedback, or speech appliances to develop appropriate placement of target sounds.

LEARNING AIDS

The format used in the book is designed to enhance student and practitioner learning:
- Each chapter begins with a **general outline** of the subject matter that is to be covered.
- Next, **key terms** are identified for the reader to provide a brief overview of the vocabulary that must be mastered to grasp the important concepts in the body of the chapter.
- The key terms are followed by specific **Learning Goals** that reflect the major treatment components of each chapter.
- A **brief chapter introduction** follows and serves to create a focus for the content of each chapter.
- **Research Notes** are incorporated in each chapter to underscore significant classic and recent advancements in the treatment literature.
- **Case studies** interspersed within chapter discussions highlight specific cases, treatments, and outcomes. Author commentary follows, with critical evaluation of the treatment and its efficacy.
- A **glossary** includes user-friendly definitions of each chapter key term and serves as a handy reference tool.

ANCILLARIES

An Evolve website (http://evolve.elsevier.com/Ruscello/articulation) provides the following resources for instructors:

- A **Test Bank** consists of approximately 200 objective-style questions—multiple-choice, true/false, and fill-in-the-blank—with accompanying rationales for correct responses and page number references to indicate where that content can be located within the textbook. Instructors may choose to use this resource to build examinations or release it to students for practice.
- An **Image Collection** features full-color electronic versions of chapter images, plus additional images that illustrate the anatomy of speech and hearing. Images can be downloaded into classroom lecture presentations or used in specific treatment situations.
- Chapter reference listings are compiled into a complete **Bibliography** with Medline links, allowing readers quick and easy reference to significant treatment literature and direct connections to specific journal articles available online.
- **Interactive flashcards** provide students with a fun and engaging way to practice vocabulary. A flashcard is provided for each term included in the glossary to help ensure content mastery.

ACKNOWLEDGMENTS

The support and encouragement of Ms. Kathy Falk during the preparation of the book is gratefully acknowledged, as is the excellent editorial assistance of Ms. Kristin Hebberd. Kristin's work and input significantly enhanced both the format and content of the book. I also want to recognize the efforts of Jonathan Taylor during the production stages of the project. I am indebted to the outstanding efforts of these individuals.

I also want to acknowledge the excellent support of my family, particularly my wife Edie.

Dennis M. Ruscello

Contents

Treating Articulation and Phonological Disorders in Children

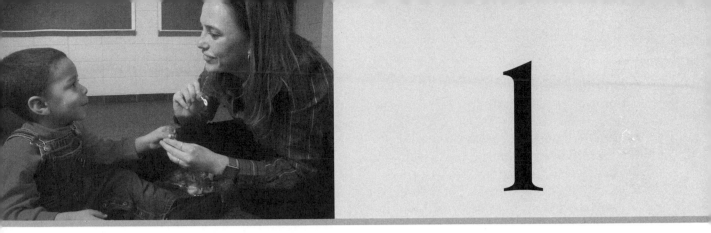

Introduction to the Treatment of Sound System Disorders

substitution errors
training trial

LEARNING GOALS ▬

- Identify several causal factors that may account for sound system disorders.
- Discuss client, clinician, and caregiver variables that must be considered in the development of any treatment plan.
- Summarize the features of both operant and motor skill–learning frameworks as they apply to articulation and phonological disorders.
- Discuss treatment factors, specifically measurement, common to both learning frameworks.

T*his introductory chapter presents the basic components of the text and serves as a guide for the reader. It will address the heterogeneous nature of sound system disorders, describe a treatment model for children with sound system disorders, and discuss general programmatic issues that must be considered in treatment. The etiology of sound system disorders is generally unknown for most children, but subgroups of children may experience structural, sensory, or neurological disorders. The differences among groups must be considered when selecting a treatment. A treatment model that attempts to incorporate all relevant treatment variables is presented as an archetype for the chapters that follow. The model incorporates child, clinician, and caregiver variables. Finally, discussion is directed to theories of learning and treatment factors that are important in planning, conducting, and evaluating treatment programs.*

The term **sound system disorder** refers to clinically significant sound production errors, which may have a phonetic or phonemic basis (Shelton, 1993). The term *sound system disorder* will be used in this text when discussing specific treatments for children who may exhibit **phonetic** (articulatory) production errors, **phonemic** (phonological) production errors, or both. The reader should note that distinctions between phonetic and phonemic disorders are difficult to establish in some cases (Kahmi, 2005), but they do represent different theoretical perspectives for understanding and treating sound system disorders (Schwartz, 1992). Moreover, the dichotomy is used in the literature to compare and contrast different treatments (Gierut, 1998). A number of terms such as *articulation disorder, delayed speech, developmental phonologic disorder, phonological disorder,* and *developmental speech sound disorder* are used in the literature (Bernthal and Bankson, 2004; Shriberg and Kwiatkowski, 1994; Williams, 2003), but *sound system disorder* will be used in this text as an inclusive classificatory term. Speech-language pathologists who work with preschool and school-aged children provide services to large numbers of children with sound system disorders of known and unknown etiology; consequently, knowledge of different treatment strategies is very important. Researchers estimate that approximately 80% of children with sound system disorders require treatment services. Moreover, about 92% of school speech-language pathologists provide services to children with sound system disorders (Castrogiovanni, 2006).

Approximately 92% of school speech-language pathologists work with children with sound system disorders.	*Research* Note

Castrogiovanni, 2006.

Shriberg and Kwiatkowski (1994) estimate that approximately 7.5% of children between 3 and 11 years of age experience clinically significant sound system disorders, and most receive treatment. For some, treatment may begin in the preschool years and continue into elementary school. The authors indicate further that about 2.5% of the group exhibit major substitution and deletion errors that continue past 4 years of age. Although some of the children in this subgroup develop normal speech, others continue to manifest substitution and deletion errors. In addition, a large proportion of the group also experience coexisting problems in the acquisition and development of reading, writing, and spelling or may be diagnosed with learning disabilities (Bird et al., 1995; Felsenfeld et al., 1994; Gierut, 1998). Moreover, some children may also demonstrate social differences as a function of their communication disorder (Rice et al., 1993). The remaining 5% of the group generally display sound errors of /s/, /l/ and /r, ɝ, ɚ/ that are classified as **residual errors** because they continue past the expected age of developmental acquisition (Ruscello, 2003). Residual errors may be remediated or continue into adulthood.

ETIOLOGY OF SOUND SYSTEM DISORDERS

Throughout the history of the profession, researchers have studied children with sound system disorders in an attempt to discover causal factors that might explain the problem (Bernthal and Bankson, 2004; Winitz, 1969). Do causal factors exist, and can they be identified? What factor or factors might account for sound system disorders? Bernthal and Bankson (2004) indicate that structural, sensory, cognitive, linguistic, and psychosocial variables have been studied extensively in an effort to discover causal factors; however, this methodology has not isolated a specific individual or group of causal agents for the majority of children with sound system disorders. As the authors point out, small subgroups of children experience sound system disorders, and these disorders are related to structural, sensory, or neurophysiologic factors (or a combination of these factors). For example, children with **structural defects** such as cleft palate have sound system disorders that are generally related to the structural problem. That is, they may frequently use **substitution errors** that are of the compensatory type, such as use of glottal stops. Hearing loss is another variable that has an adverse effect on phonological development. **Motor speech disorders** that are related to motor planning or central and peripheral neurological problems also exist in a small subgroup of children with sound system disorders. Because definitive causal factors have not been identified for the large majority of children with sound system disorders, researchers have also tried to identify causal correlates or a cluster of variables that may coexist with sound system disorders; however, no definite cluster has been identified to date. Bernthal and Bankson conclude that practitioners must have an understanding of variables related to sound system disorders to assess, treat, and counsel the caregivers of children with sound system disorders.

Table 1-1 is a summary classification of children with sound system disorders. Most children who receive treatment services have sound system disorders of unknown origin. That is, no single causal factor or causal correlates have been identified with this group of children—the cause is attributed to mislearning. However, children with structural defects frequently exhibit sound errors related to the defect (Golding-Kushner, 2001; Peterson-Falzone, 1988). Structural anomalies may include conditions such as cleft lip and palate, jaw malocclusion, tongue malformations, and missing teeth. Another subgroup of children with sound system disorders includes children with sensory deficits such as hearing loss (Ling, 2002; Paterson, 1994). Hearing is an important sensory modality, and hearing loss can significantly affect both

Table 1-1
Classification of Children with Sound System Disorders

SOUND SYSTEM DISORDER	CAUSAL VARIABLE
No identifiable causal factor	Unknown origin
Oral structural defect	Major and minor oral anomalies
Sensory deficit	Type and degree of hearing loss

Motor speech disorders
    Apraxia
    Dysarthria
	Motor planning, motor execution
	    disorders, or both

speech and language development. Finally, motor speech disorders may result from some type of neurological problem (Yorkston et al., 1999). The problem may manifest in motor planning, coordination of muscle movement, timing of movements, implementation of the movement patterns requisite to normal speech production, or a combination of these factors. In addition to an articulatory component, a motor speech disorder may also include involvement of other biocommunication systems such as respiration, phonation, resonation, and speech prosody.

TO SUM UP

Previously cited statistics indicate that many practitioners provide treatment services to children with sound system disorders. Furthermore, most children exhibit sound system disorders of unknown etiology, but low-incidence subgroups with explicit causes are seen. These data indicate that the typical caseload of the practitioner who provides services to children with sound system disorders will consist mainly of children with problems of unknown etiology. The practitioner needs to have the knowledge and skills to treat these children but must also be knowledgeable and skilled in the treatment of low-incidence populations. This requires facility with a variety of treatment strategies that vary as a function of phonological behavior and the presence of causal factors. In her seminal review of treatment studies, Gierut (1998) concludes that various treatments for sound system disorders, which represent different theoretical perspectives, have demonstrated positive results. The treatments are effective, but a host of factors come into play during the treatment process. That is, client, practitioner, and caregiver variables need to be considered because of their potential influence on the treatment process. In the next section, a framework or model will be discussed that can be used in the treatment of sound system disorders.

Research Note	A variety of treatments based on varying theoretical perspectives have yielded positive results in children with sound system disorders.

Gierut, 1998.

PROPOSED TREATMENT MODEL

The **National Outcome Measurement System (NOMS)** is a project that is being conducted by the American Speech-Language-Hearing Association (ASHA) for the purpose of collecting treatment data on speech and language disorders. (ASHA members can access more information on this project directly at www.asha.org.) Preliminary findings indicate that more positive outcomes for sound system disorders are found for young children who receive individual versus group therapy, are enrolled for 10 or more hours of treatment, and have a caregiver conduct home treatment practice. The positive outcome occurred despite the use of different treatments (which likely differed according to theoretical rationale and application). However, common components included the fact that treatments were carried out individually, a sufficient period of time was allotted for treatment, and practitioners enlisted the aid of caregivers in all cases. In selecting a treatment, clinicians should consider a number of different treatment variables regardless of the theory that underlies their treatment of sound system disorders (Schwartz, 1992).

Research Note	Children with sound system disorders who receive individual therapy for 10 or more hours and who have a caregiver practicing in-home treatment benefit most from treatment.

American Speech-Language-Hearing Association, 2006.

Box 1-1 presents a proposed treatment model that reflects client, clinician, and caregiver variables (Bowen and Cupples, 2004; Gierut, 1998; Kwiatkowski and Shriberg, 1998; Munson et al., 2005a; Rvachew, 2005;

BOX 1-1   *Variables Incorporated into a Treatment Framework for Sound System Disorders*

Client, clinician, and caregiver variables all affect treatment selection and are outlined as follows:

Client Variables

Client Status
Stimulability
Self-monitoring skills
Effort of the client
Attention of the client
Motivation of the client for change
Treatment history
Interactions with clinician and caregiver

Phonological Knowledge
Acoustic and phonetic knowledge
Articulatory and phonetic knowledge
Internal phonological knowledge

Potential Risk Factors
Cognitive and linguistic status
Speech mechanism
Hearing acuity
Neurophysiologic status

Clinician Variables
Knowledge and skills
Theoretical biases
Confidence in treatment
Interactions with client and caregiver

Caregiver Variables
Confidence in clinician
Confidence in treatment
Willingness to assist in treatment
Interactions with client and clinician

Weiss, 2004). The hypothetical model is the author's interpretation of the seminal work of Kwiatkowski and Shriberg (1998) and Rvachew (2005), who suggest that an adequate treatment model must consider **cognitive-linguistic variables, motor skill learning,** phonological knowledge, social skills, and a number of potential risk factors. This archetype is proposed for client treatment regardless of the treatment and its underlying theoretical rationale.

Research Note	An adequate treatment model must consider cognitive-linguistic variables, motor skill learning, phonological knowledge, social skills, and potential risk factors.

Kwiatkowski and Shriberg, 1998; Rvachew, 2005.

Client Variables

The major client categories of the proposed model include client status, phonological knowledge, and risk variables. The variables are derived primarily from the **capability-focus construct** proposed by Kwaitkowski and Shriberg (1998). Capability is the capacity or potential of the child for speech change as determined through assessment of the child's phonology and the consideration of any presenting risk factors. Focus is a hypothetical construct that incorporates the learning requisites of attention, motivation, and effort. Stimulability and self-monitoring skills are client status variables that reflect both capability and focus. Additional client status variables are the treatment history of the client and the interaction of the client with the clinician and caregiver. Client status variables are important considerations when analyzing the results of an assessment, planning treatment, and monitoring the child's performance to the treatment. It should be noted that any of the client status variables could be a strength or weakness for the child (Figure 1-1). For example, deficient self-monitoring skills may be identified during assessment and need to be targeted in treatment, or the monitoring of training trails indicates a lack of learning that may require an alteration in treatment to improve the client's response to remediation.

Phonological knowledge is the person's knowledge of the sound system of a language. During communication development, the child gradually acquires this knowledge. Phonological knowledge is a composite of acoustic and perceptual knowledge, articulatory and phonetic knowledge, and internal phonological knowledge (Munson et al., 2005a). The child with a sound system disorder is delayed in the acquisition of phonological knowledge and requires some form of treatment to develop intelligible speech. During development the child acquires knowledge of the acoustic and perceptual features of the language through auditory input from a variety of speakers in the environment. The child's goal is to develop knowledge of the acoustic and perceptual characteristics of

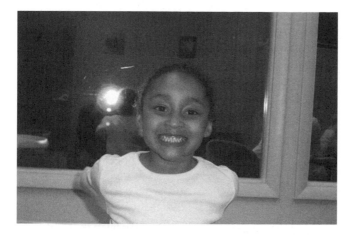

Figure 1-1 ■ Clients who are interested and motivated to change their sound system errors are positive candidates for treatment.

different word shapes and the acceptable boundaries of within-class sound production that is a function of categorical perception. **Articulatory knowledge** is the child's knowledge of the production features of sounds. A competent speaker must have motor-planning strategies that allow correct sound production across a range of sound combinations and in a variety of speaking tasks. **Internal phonological knowledge** is knowledge of the ways that sound categories are used to signal meaning differences and permissible ways that the sound categories are used in word construction. Munson et al. (2005b) provide preliminary evidence to support the position that sound system disorders are related primarily to acoustic-perceptual and articulatory-phonetic problems, not internal phonological knowledge. That is, children with phonological disorders appear to experience more difficulty in the sensory and motor domains, rather than mapping abstract representations of items in their lexicons; however, the preliminary data require further empirical validation.

Researchers believe that sound system disorders are related primarily to acoustic-perceptual and articulatory-phonetic problems, as opposed to internal phonological knowledge.

Research Note

Munson et al., 2005b.

Risk factors are potential constraints that may adversely affect speech and influence a child's treatment regimen. Unlike client status variables, which may be positive or negative factors, risk factors are concerns that need to be considered in developing a treatment plan. For example, cognitive-linguistic status is a problem for some children because they may have a coexisting speech or language impairment that also requires treatment (Tyler and Sandoval, 1994). The coexistence of speech sound disorders with other speech and language disorders is quite substantial, particularly in the population of children with severe sound system disorders (Shriberg, 1994; St. Louis et al., 1992). Speech mechanism variables such as missing teeth, malocclusion, cleft palate, and other problems may be causal agents in the development and maintenance of compensatory and obligatory sound system disorders (Golding-Kushner, 2001; Peterson-Falzone, 1988). Similarly, hearing acuity and neurophysiologic status are additional risk variables that must be considered because they may interfere with the acquisition of acoustic-phonetic and articulatory-phonetic knowledge (see Box 1-1).

Clinician Variables

Although generally not considered in reporting and advocating for different treatments, clinician variables are an integral part of the proposed treatment model (Weiss, 2004). A practitioner has acquired a certain amount of knowledge regarding the management of children with sound system disorders through academic coursework, continuing education, self-study, and interaction with colleagues. The knowledge has been applied during graduate education and professional practice so that the practitioner has developed certain skills, which are applied in the treatment process. Skills such as implementing a specific treatment, developing a child's stimulability skills, evaluating client responses, monitoring progress, and making alterations to a treatment are just a few examples of the skills used by practitioners in their daily practice. The knowledge and skills are subsumed into the practitioner's theory of clinical practice.

Schwartz (1992) points out that, consciously or unconsciously, practitioners operate under a theory that influences what they do therapeutically and how they do it. However, the practitioner must remain conscious of underlying theory because it will allow the implementation of a treatment in a systematic fashion. Moreover, clinical practice will change as more comprehensive theories of clinical practice are formulated, and the practitioner must be sensitive to such change (Kamhi, 1999). Confidence in a treatment is a union of the practitioner's theoretical assumptions and experience with that particular treatment.

Caregiver Variables

The final variable—one that is common to all parties of the proposed model—is that of social interaction. Generally an implicit goal of treatment is to establish a positive clinical interaction with the child and caregiver. Weiss (2004) indicates that the development of a positive relationship is achieved through the establishment of rapport, which she believes is often overlooked in the therapy situation. **Rapport** is the establishment of a supportive relationship between the practitioner and child as well as the practitioner and parent. Weiss believes that rapport is something that must be maintained throughout the treatment period, because rapport is a factor that is associated with positive treatment outcomes.

Parents also play an important role in the treatment of their children in terms of both attitude toward treatment and willingness to assist in the treatment process. Kahmi (1999) points out that caregivers must have confidence in the clinician and the treatment that is to be used because caregivers are interested in the welfare of their children. They have sought the guidance of a clinician, or a clinician has contacted them because of the child's sound system disorder. Caregivers need to be reassured that the clinician is acting in the best interests of the child. In addition to attitudinal variables, parents are often asked to assist with treatment by conducting home practice sessions; their willingness to participate actively in the therapeutic process is a positive factor (Bowen and Cupples, 1999, 2004). Caregiver interest, support, and participation are generally positive factors. However, instances occur when caregiver interactions are not positive, and the result may negatively influence the intended treatment outcome. For example, if a caregiver is too demanding of the child during home practice, then home activities may need to be curtailed.

The model was designed to assist practitioners in selecting and implementing a treatment that is consistent with the child's needs. The clinician must choose a treatment from a number of treatment options (based on the client variables that were discussed). The clinician should base the treatment on what the child needs, not what the clinician is comfortable doing. The next section deals with treatment factors that are the basis for implementing a treatment. They constitute the mechanics of treatment—the *how* of conducting treatment for children with sound system disorders.

TREATMENT FACTORS

The first consideration in treatment is to organize instructional objectives within a theoretical learning framework for the purpose of client learning. Current conceptualizations of the treatment of sound system disorders generally use either operant learning or a motor skill–learning framework for treatment (Bernthal and Bankson, 2004). Both theoretical treatment frameworks have been subject to extensive empirical scrutiny, and findings support the validity of each in the treatment of sound system disorders (Costello, 1977; Gierut, 1998; Hedge, 1993; Ruscello, 1993). Practitioners must be aware of the major features of each learning framework so that a treatment may be applied within the bounds of the theory. In the clinical literature, an operant framework has been used in the treatment of both phonetic- and phonemic-based disorders, whereas a motor skill–learning rationale has generally been used for phonetic-based disorders (Bernthal and Bankson, 2004).

Research Note   An operant learning framework has been used to structure treatment for both phonetic- and phonemic-based disorders. A motor skill–learning model has been used to treat phonetic-based disorders.

Bernthal and Bankson, 2004.

Operant Learning

The instructional cycle of stimulus-response-reinforcement is the hallmark of **operant learning** (Bernthal and Bankson, 2004). Stimuli or **antecedent events** are used to evoke specific responses from the client. **Consequent events** immediately follow the response and are used to either reinforce a response behavior or punish in the case of an unwanted behavior. The treatment of sound system disorders generally involves the use of positive reinforcers so that the likelihood of the child developing a class of desired responses is increased (Costello, 1977). Generally the clinician ignores incorrect responses or the verbal "no" is used, after which a new stimulus is provided. Reinforcers may be categorized as either *primary* or *secondary reinforcers*. **Primary reinforcers** are directed to biological or physiological needs (or to both), such as the use of food to reinforce desired behavior. **Secondary reinforcers** are selected because they are of intrinsic value to the learner. Young clients are frequently motivated to achieve the goals of treatment and change their phonological performance. Often practitioners use secondary reinforcers such as verbal praise, token economies, and performance feedback to stimulate learning (Hedge, 1993). Another important aspect of reinforcement is the schedule or frequency with which the reinforcement is provided to the learner. Generally reinforcement is provided on a continuous basis during the early stages of learning, but shifts to intermittent delivery when the client begins to show that learning is occurring. Learned behaviors are more resistant to extinction under intermittent reinforcement than under continuous reinforcement (Costello, 1977). Moreover, intermittent reinforcement is a closer approximation to the natural environment, which the clinician is trying to achieve through treatment to foster generalization.

Learned behaviors tend to be more resistant to extinction under intermittent reinforcement as opposed to continuous reinforcement.

Research Note

Costello, 1977.

The reader should note that the learning of a new behavior and the rate of that learning are intrinsically related to the consequent events (reinforcers) that follow the desired response (Bernthal and Bankson, 2004). Accordingly, the clinician needs to consider carefully the reinforcer that is to be used with a specific client, because individual clients may respond differently to a specific reinforcer. Once the response class has been established in treatment, the clinician will shift from continuous to intermittent reinforcement; this is because the ultimate goal is the generalization of phonetic and/or phonemic behavior to the child's natural environment.

In a typical treatment paradigm, the clinician implements stimulus-cueing procedures to promote the learning of specific communicative responses. Different stimulus cues are used at different stages of the learning process. For example, Costello (1977) points out that early learning is characterized by the use of various cues, prompts, and different models. These stimulus cues are gradually eliminated in favor of cues that are related to the projected outcome or terminal goal of the treatment. The following examples, which are summarized in Box 1-2, illustrate some of the different stimulus-cueing techniques that may be introduced in treatment. The first example is imitation, which is frequently used during the initial stages of treatment and then gradually eliminated. Shaping is the second technique and consists of isolating the components of a behavior, teaching the components individually, and

---

BOX 1-2   *Stimulus-Cueing Techniques in Operant Learning*

Imitation
Used during initial stages and usually eliminated

Shaping
Isolating behavior components, teaching them individually, and incorporating the behaviors to attain the desired response

Prompts
Usually paired with a specific set of stimuli; can be attentional (for client focus) or instructional (to facilitate correct responses)

Fading or Shifting
Used when a training step has been mastered; specific cue is replaced by another cue

---

then incorporating the behaviors to attain the desired response. In the example, the child first learns jaw, lip, and tongue postures as requisite to production of /s/. After mastery, the postures are combined with the actual production of the target. The third example is a prompt; the purpose is to provide further support to the client. Prompts are usually paired with a specific set of stimuli, and they can be either attentional or instructional. Attentional prompts are designed to create additional client focus by asking the child to observe the clinician or both observe and listen to the stimulus being presented. Instructional prompts are used to facilitate correct responses through the use of instructions regarding placement of the articulators or cautioning the client about the production features of the error sound. The final example is that of fading or shifting stimulus cues when a training step has been mastered. In this case, the clinician uses a specific stimulus cue to replace another one as illustrated in the sequence. The initial response was that of imitation, followed by imitation paired with a picture, and finally presentation of the picture alone to elicit a spontaneous response.

The examples in Table 1-2 illustrate different ways of eliciting responses during the initial stages of treatment when the goal is to establish the targets in a nucleus of words. However, it may be necessary to shift to other stimuli that will facilitate the production of targets in practice stimuli, such as phrases, sentences, and spontaneous conversation. The use of such a progression suggests that less complex linguistic material must be mastered before more complex material. Nevertheless,

Table 1-2
Examples of Training Trials within an Operant Learning Paradigm

STIMULUS	RESPONSE	REINFORCEMENT
Direct Imitation "Say each word after me." "Say the word *soup*."	"Soup."	"Good job!"

"I'll show you a picture and
  say the word for you. Then
  say it. Ready, say the word
  soup."
	"Soup."	"Great!"

Shaping
"We're going to learn to
  make the /s/ sound. First, I
  want you to smile and watch
  yourself in the mirror. Let's do
  it together now."
	Client smiles with the lips apart
	  and incisors closed
		"That's good!"

"This time we're going to
  do the same thing, but now
  we're also going to blow some
  air off the tongue. Remember
  to keep your tongue behind
  your front teeth."
	Client smiles with the lips apart
	  and incisors approximated
	  and makes the /s/
		"Good."

Prompting
"I'm going to show you a
  picture, and I want you to tell
  me a short story about it.
  Remember to look at me when
  you're talking!"
	Client looks at clinician and
	  verbalizes the request
		"Good talking!"

"I want you to make your
  new sound in the words that
  I'll show you. Remember to
  keep your tongue from
  sticking out!"
	Client produces the target
	  correctly
		"Very good!"

Continued

Table 1-2
Examples of Training Trials within an Operant Learning Paradigm—cont'd

STIMULUS	RESPONSE	REINFORCEMENT
Fading Clinician presents direct imitative model and asks the child to say it.	Client responds	"Good."
Clinician presents direct imitative model and pairs it with a picture of the practice item.	Client responds	"Good."
Clinician presents a picture and asks the client to produce the item.	Client responds	"Good."

the practitioner must remember that the instructional cycle of stimulus-response-reinforcement must be carefully applied so that maximum learning is achieved, and taught behaviors generalize to the natural environment.

Motor Skill Learning

Researchers have applied theoretical models of motor skill learning to the treatment of children with sound system disorders (Kent and Lybolt, 1982; Ruscello, 1984; Ruscello, 1993; Shelton and McReynolds, 1979). Although operant learning has been applied to the modification of a number of different speech and nonspeech behaviors, motor skill–learning theory and performance principles have been developed to teach simple and complex motor skills (Schmidt and Wrisberg, 2000). Researchers theorize that the learner passes through different stages of motor skill development when engaged in formal practice (Ruscello, 1984). Initially the learner attempts to acquire a motor skill through activities that incorporate practice under conscious control. That is, the learner needs to "think" about what he or she is practicing. Higgins (1991) writes that the learner is placed in a problem-solving situation that requires mental focus during the initial stages of practice. The motor skill is carried out in a restricted, self-guided mode with feedback and **knowledge of results (KR)** provided by the clinician. **Feedback** is information the learner internalizes from practice trials through various forms of sensory feedback and conscious introspection, whereas KR is performance information provided by an external source such as the clinician. The KR can be qualitative ("Good job!") or quantitative ("Your tongue was sticking out!"), or both.

Operant learning has been applied to the modification of a number of speech and nonspeech behaviors, whereas motor skill–learning theory and performance principles have been developed to teach simple and complex motor skills such as sound production.

Research Note

Schmidt and Wrisberg, 2000.

The examples in Table 1-3 provide the reader with insight regarding the structuring of treatment activities. In the first example the clinician provides the client with sound placement instructions and an imitative model, evaluates the response, and provides qualitative KR information. Feedback information that the learner internalizes from the practice trial is also available for processing by the client. The second example is similar to the first in that the clinician provides an imitative model but does not include placement instructions. After the response, KR is provided. In the third example the clinician elicits a spontaneous response from the client using picture stimuli. Both quantitative and qualitative KR are provided after the correct response is given. The final example depicts the use of a nonce item. A **nonce item** is a sound combination that is not a morpheme, and it may or may not have a permissible phonological structure. Generally, a nonce item is paired with a picture or line drawing to associate meaning with the nonce item. The underlying rationale is to have the child practice a "word unit," which is not in his or her lexicon to reduce interference from the error response. The item is presented as the shape illustrated and is not phonologically permissible.

Practice is an important aspect of motor skill learning, and different types of practice are used at different stages of treatment (Schmidt and Wrisberg, 2000). After the learner has acquired the skill through practice and conscious introspection, additional practice activities are introduced to automate the skilled pattern (Ruscello, 1993). The learner no longer

Table 1-3
Examples of Training Trials within a Motor Skill–Learning Paradigm

CLINICIAN'S PRESENTATION	LEARNER'S RESPONSE	FEEDBACK/KR
Placement Instructions/Imitation "I want you to think about your new sound in the word. Remember to put your tongue behind your teeth for the /s/. Think about where you are putting your tongue and then say the word."	"soap"	"Good job!" (KR)
Imitative Response Elicitation "Say the name of each picture after I say it." "Say the word _____."	"soap"	"Good." (KR)
Quantitative/Qualitative Feedback "I'll show you a picture, and I want you to say it."	"soap"	"Good job." (KR) "You made your tongue work and kept it behind your teeth." (KR)
Use of Nonce Items "This is a /sri/." ⬭ "Say /sri/."	"sri"	"Good job!" (KR)

KR, Knowledge of result.

needs to focus on the mental substrates of the skill but rather carries out the skill under a variety of conditions and practice contexts. The skill is becoming part of the learner's motor skill repertoire. Research suggests that distributed practice of a motor skill results in slightly better learning and retention than massed practice. For example, one would predict that three 20-minute sessions spread across 1 week would be more effective than a single, weekly, 60-minute session.

Similar to operant learning, motor skill–learning treatment generally consists of a stairstep strategy, which progresses from isolation to conversational practice. Isolation, nonce or nonsense words, words, phrases, sentences, and conversational speech are used as judged necessary by the clinician. Under the guise of motor learning, the progression of practice material is presented in two different ways: block sequencing or random sequencing. **Block sequencing** is most typical with material introduced in stairstep order as discussed. For example, a child achieves correct target production in words and is then exposed to phrases. **Random sequencing** is different in that the child is exposed to the practice of all conditions in a random sequence during a treatment session (Skelton, 2004). For example, a random presentation of practice material that ranges from syllables to conversation is introduced randomly in a single session. The child may first practice sentences, followed by words and then conversation. Research suggests that random sequencing results in slightly lower accuracy rates during practice sessions than block sequencing; however, greater generalization to nontrained items occurs with random sequencing (Schmidt and Wrisberg, 2000; Skelton, 2004).

According to research, random sequencing shows a slightly lower accuracy rate than block sequencing during practice sessions, but generalization to nontrained items is greater with random sequencing.

Research Note

Schmidt and Wrisberg, 2000; Skelton, 2004.

TO SUM UP

The clinician may provide treatment under either of the theoretical frameworks described. The selection will, of course, depend on the sound system disorder that the client exhibits. Each framework is somewhat different in terms of procedure but not in process, because both share the ultimate goal of increased learning. Table 1-4 contrasts the two theoretical models in relation to eight different features. Inspection shows similarities in terms of application and the use of different prompts and cues to facilitate correct sound production. The major difference between the two learning theories is the inclusion of mental practice features. Motor skill learning places more emphasis on the cognitive aspect of sound production skill. Clients are asked to focus mentally on the motor task during the initial stages of skill development and use introspection to acquire the desired movement pattern. Operant learn-

Table 1-4 Contrast of the Two Theoretical Approaches	
OPERANT LEARNING	**MOTOR LEARNING**
Used in applications of both phonemic and phonetic treatment	Used in applications of phonetic treatment
Does not include stages of response development	Includes stages of response development that correspond to levels of skill control; acquisition is followed by automatization
Treatment is conducted within the instructional cycle of stimulus-response-reinforcement	Treatment is conducted within the instructional cycle of stimulus-response-feedback/KR
Does not emphasize mental focus on sound production features	Emphasizes mental focus on sound production features, particularly during the early stages of response development
Uses a variety of different cues and prompts to elicit responses	Uses a variety of different cues and prompts to elicit responses
May use a stairstep strategy to introduce different levels of linguistic practice material	May use a stairstep strategy (block) or random presentation to introduce different levels of linguistic practice material
Does not use mental rehearsal	May use mental rehearsal of a skill after it has been acquired
Used as a learning framework to restructure the phonological system	Used as a learning framework to teach motor skills requisite to sound production

KR, Knowledge of results.

ing is more a "means to an end" in phonemic treatment, because this type of learning is used to present phonemic contrasts in a systematic and efficient way. The phonemic contrasts are designed to create change in the client's internalized phonemic system.

COMMON TREATMENT FACTORS

When using either theoretical learning approach, the clinician needs to know how to teach, what to teach, and when the child has met the goal of treatment. This will require a number of clinical decisions by the clinician and, when appropriate, in cooperation with the client and the client's caregivers. This section addresses a number of common treatment issues, regardless of the theoretical teaching framework that is used. The common issues will deal with the measurement of client performance and the activities that are used in treatment.

Measurement of Treatment

Olswang and Bain (1994) identified the following four important clinical measurement variables used to validate a treatment effect:
1. Child's response to treatment
2. Amount of change associated with treatment
3. Establishment of a treatment effect
4. Determination of length of treatment
   To measure change, quantitative and qualitative data need to be collected before, during, and after treatment. The different categories of data are treatment data, generalization probe data, and control data. Each type of quantitative data needs to be defined operationally so that the clinician can actually measure the variables of interest.

Training Trials

Treatment data consist of the responses of the client during individual treatment sessions (Olswang and Bain, 1994). Each **training trial** is evaluated for accuracy; records of the client's response accuracy percentages are maintained for each therapy activity, as well as information regarding his or her overall performance in each session. For example, a client may practice words with the target sound in the prevocalic position under the successive conditions of imitation, imitation paired with a picture, and the picture alone during a treatment session. The clinician needs to determine whether (1) the child has mastered an individual treatment condition and the next treatment condition should be introduced or (2) the treatment condition is too difficult for the child and must be reintroduced or modified. This is achieved by using some form of pass criterion (i.e., what the child must achieve before changing a treatment condition). Traditionally, clinicians set high accuracy levels that range from 80% to 90%, and the percentages are set for a specified number of training trials or period of time. For instance, the client may need to achieve an accuracy level of 90% for 20 consecutive training trials or correctly produce two consecutive blocks of 8 of 10 correct responses. A time-passing criterion might be 80% accuracy of an individual treatment condition in a 15-minute period of treatment. Achievement of the pass criterion signals the completion of a treatment goal and the introduction of a new goal. If measurable criteria are not set, determining progression within a treatment strategy is difficult.

Research Note	Treatment performance data consist of client responses during individual treatment sessions.

Olswang and Bain, 1994.

The clinician also needs to establish the overall response accuracy percentage to quantify the child's performance for that therapy session. The rationale is to examine the client's session-by-session achievement to ensure that the therapy goals are being met. As with the individual treatment conditions, overall session accuracy percentages would be expected in the range of 80% to 90%. If response data dip below criterion levels, then the clinician needs to evaluate the treatment and implement necessary changes so that learning is occurring. Clinicians must be cognizant of the fact that the response data must be unambiguous to be scored. They should use a dichotomous scale so that perceptual qualifiers such as "that was close" are avoided. Olswang and Bain (1994) point out that supplemental qualitative data also may be obtained by subjective judgment of the child's motivation and effort—what Kwiatkowski and Shriberg (1998) have identified as *focus*. The collection of treatment data is one way to monitor the client's learning in regard to the actual teaching conditions, but it does not provide information on the use of treatment targets outside of therapy (Baker and McLeod, 2004).

Assessment of Generalization

The client's performance on generalization measures provides information on the extension of learning outside of therapy and can be monitored through the use of a single-subject design (Williams, 1993). That is, the clinician wants to verify that the child is using the treatment targets outside of the therapy in naturalistic contexts (Baker and McLeod, 2004). Generally the clinician assesses stimulus generalization and response generalization. **Stimulus generalization** examines the use of actual treatment exemplars in nontreatment contexts or with individuals who are not involved with the treatment, such as caregivers. For example, the client may begin to use some actual training exemplars in his or her classroom, indicating that the learning is extending beyond the treatment context. **Response generalization** is the extension of targets to untrained items and response classes (generally assessed through the use of probes within the single-subject design). The purpose is to collect response data on the target, the response class of the target, or situational contexts not receiving treatment (Bain and Dollaghan, 1991). For example, a client may have an /s/ production error that is being treated. Before treatment and periodically during treatment, the clinician administers a probe of 20 items that contain pictures depicting words, phrases, and sentences with the target sound. These items are not taught in treatment. The client is shown the pictures and spontaneously responds to each; he or she is not given feedback regarding performance. The clinician evaluates each response and tabulates the data to determine whether the child is generalizing. If the accuracy of the probes increases with treatment, then the clinician can conclude that the treatment has a positive effect because the client is beginning to use the target in untreated exemplars. Additional confidence in the treatment may also be demonstrated by including a withdrawal component. The treatment is withdrawn, and response generalization should show a stable pattern of performance or a decrement in performance. Subjective data may be obtained by caregiver reports of the client using the target in new words and with other individuals.

Bain and Dollaghan (1991) indicate that additional confidence in a treatment can be obtained by including a **control behavior** within the single-subject design. A control behavior is a behavior that is independent from the behavior that is subject to treatment. In the previous example, /s/ was the sound selected for treatment. If the child misarticulated the /r/ sound, then it could be used as a control sound because it differs from /s/ in a number of phonetic production features. One would predict a change in /s/ with treatment and no change in production of /r/ because it was not the target of therapy and is phonetically dissimilar to /s/.

The inclusion of a control behavior within a single-subject design can provide the clinician with additional confidence in a treatment.

Research Note

Bain and Dollaghan, 1991.

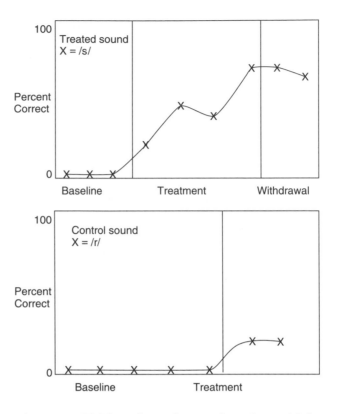

Figure 1-2 ■ Hypothetical examples of a multiple baseline showing treated and control sounds. This fictitious client has both /s/ and /r/ errors.

Figure 1-2 shows a hypothetical case of a client who has both /s/ and /r/ errors. The treatment target is /s/ and is depicted in the first graph. The baseline, or pretherapy, measure shows three sampling points that are stable and show no recorded correct responses. The baseline pattern indicates that /s/ is a valid target for treatment. Treatment is instituted, and a positive change is seen in response generalization. The treatment is then withdrawn, and the generalization probes demonstrate a decrement in performance. This pattern of response generalization suggests that the treatment was responsible for the change noted. Further confidence in the treatment is present in the second graph that summarizes the hypothetical /r/ data. A stable baseline is maintained at all sampling points. Positive change in /s/ is noted, but there is no change in /r/ until treatment is instituted. At that time an increase in /r/ productions is noted, indicating that treatment of /r/ is having a positive effect

Table 1-5 **Formulae for Computing Different Types of Comparison Data**	
Percentage of correct target behaviors	$\dfrac{\text{Number of target behaviors} \times 100}{\text{Number of target opportunities}}$
Frequency of occurrence	$\dfrac{\text{Number of intervals target occurred} \times 100}{\text{Total number of intervals}}$
Rate of occurrence	$\dfrac{\text{Number of target behaviors}}{\text{Unit of time}}$
Duration of occurrence	$\dfrac{\text{Time of target behaviors} \times 100}{\text{Total observational time}}$

on /r/. The /r/ speech sound serves as a control for /s/ and further supports the /s/ treatment. The single-subject design is an effective yet simple clinical tool that the clinician can use to demonstrate positive change of a client's sound system.

In most cases of data collection for sound system disorders, the percentage of correct target behaviors is used to describe performance; however, Williams (1993) indicates that other forms of data may be used, such as the frequency of occurrence, the rate of occurrence, and the duration of occurrence. For instance, the clinician may need to chart a target behavior during predetermined time intervals, thus providing information on the frequency of occurrence of the target behavior across the time intervals. The rate of occurrence is the ratio between the number of times that the target behavior was used within a predetermined amount of time. Finally, the duration of occurrence is a measure that compares the time of occurrence of a target behavior in relation to the total time of observation. Table 1-5 provides summary descriptions of the formulae for computing the various measures.

Treatment Activities

All treatment programs use different client activities to facilitate production of treatment targets. Shriberg and Kwiatkowski (1982) conducted a comprehensive literature review and indicate that client treatment activities consist mainly of drill, drill/play, structured play, and play. **Drill** is the presentation of stimuli without the benefit of some preceding motivational action or activity for the client. The rationale is to facilitate the elicitation of many responses in a highly repetitive manner so that treatment is maximized. **Drill/play** differs from drill in that some motivational action or activity is the antecedent. Motivational events are designed to facilitate learning by improving the client's attention and increasing learning opportunities. For example, a child may be instructed to select a picture item of choice among practice items or take a turn with a spinner game and then produce the target. Shriberg and Kwiatkowski indicate that **structured play** is similar to drill/play, but the treatment activity is carried out in a play environment that is interesting and pleasurable to the child. The play interactions are organized to elicit target responses from the client, particularly if the child experiences problems with the structure of the drill and it becomes necessary to shift to structured play. The final category is that of **naturalistic play** or what the child perceives as play. The different play activities are designed to elicit the desired target responses. The clinician may use different elicitation techniques such as self-talk and modeling to promote the production of target responses in a more naturalistic setting.

Research Note	Client treatment activities consist of (1) drill, (2) drill/play, (3) structured play, and (4) play. Of the four, drill and drill/play were found to be equally superior to structured play and play in terms of effectiveness and efficiency.

Shriberg and Kwiatkowski, 1982.

Shriberg and Kwiatkowski (1982) carried out three different investigations to examine the four different client activities. They found that drill and drill/play were superior to structured play or play in terms of effectiveness and efficiency, and no advantage was found between the effectiveness and efficiency of drill and drill/play. The clinicians who participated in the studies favored drill/play as the most effective and efficient of the treatment activities.

Terminal Goal

A final common element to be discussed is that of the terminal goal for the client. The terminal goal is that level of response production projected by the clinician before the initiation of treatment (Costello, 1977). What level of response performance is appropriate for the client at the termination of treatment? The goal is established on the basis of diagnostic testing and the treatment philosophy of the clinician. Regardless, it needs to be defined operationally so that it can be measured. Pipe (1966) emphasizes the need for the clinician to establish a realistic goal that can be measured easily. For instance, one could set a terminal goal for treatment of /s/. The client would meet the terminal goal when achieving an accuracy rate of 90% for /s/ tokens in a 10-minute sample of spontaneous conversational speech. A terminal goal may not be achieved in all instances, but it provides a guide to develop appropriate treatment activities and to gauge the improvement of the client.

SUMMARY

Children with sound system disorders constitute a heterogeneous group of individuals, and the clinician must have the appropriate knowledge and skills to treat them. Although a majority has sound system disorders of unknown etiology, subgroups of clients exist who exhibit structural, sensory, or neurological causal factors (or a combination of these factors). The differences among groups must be taken into account in the selection and application of a particular treatment. To consider all relevant variables, a treatment model is proposed as a guide for clinicians (and as an organizational framework for discussion of the different treatments covered in the book). The model considers client, clinician, and caregiver variables. In addition, theoretical explanations of learning as applied to sound system disorders are discussed in relation to their major features. The theoretical constructs are also compared and contrasted for the reader. Operant learning is used as a teaching framework to confront the child with phonemic contrasts in a systematic and efficient manner. Motor skill–learning theory is used as a teaching framework to teach sound production skills in a systematic and efficient manner. Finally, treatment factors that are common to both learning theories are discussed. The common treatment factors are used to measure objectively the client's response to the treatment. This chapter serves as the foundation for the other chapters, which deal with general treatment strategies and treatment strategies that have been developed for specific subgroups of children with sound system disorders.

REFERENCES

American Speech-Language-Hearing Association: *Pre-Kindergarten NOMS Fact Sheet: Preschoolers with articulation disorders—what affects progress?* Rockville, Md, 2006, American Speech-Language-Hearing Association.

Bain BA, Dollaghan CA: The notion of clinically significant change, *Lang Speech Hear Serv Sch* 22:264-270, 1991.

Baker E, McLeod S: Evidence-based management of phonological impairment in children, *Child Lang Teach Ther* 20:261-285, 2004.

Bernthal JE, Bankson NW: *Articulation and phonological disorders,* ed 5, Boston, 2004, Allyn & Bacon.

Bird J, Bishop DVM, Freeman NH: Phonological awareness and literacy development in children with expressive phonological impairment, *J Speech Hear Res* 38:446-462, 1995.

Bowen C, Cupples L: Parents and children together (PACT): a collaborative approach to phonological therapy, *Int J Lang Commun Disord* 34:35-83, 1999.

Bowen C, Cupples L: The role of families in optimizing phonological therapy outcomes, *Child Lang Teach Ther* 20:245-260, 2004.

Castrogiovanni A: *Communication facts: incidence and prevalence of communication disorders and hearing loss in children,* Rockville, Md, 2006, American Speech-Language-Hearing Association. Available at: www.asha. org/members/research/reports/children. Accessed September 2, 2006.

Costello JM: Programmed instruction, *J Speech Hear Disord* 42:3-28, 1977.

Felsenfeld S, Broen PA, McGue M: A 28-year follow-up of adults with a history of moderate phonological disorder: educational and occupational results, *J Speech Hear Res* 37:1341-1353, 1994.

Gierut JA: Treatment efficacy: functional phonological disorders in children, *J Speech Lang Hear Res* 41(1):S85-S100, 1998.

Golding-Kushner KJ: *Therapy techniques for cleft palate speech and related disorders,* San Diego, 2001, Singular.

Hedge MN: *Treatment procedures in communicative disorders,* ed 2, Austin, Tex, 1993, Pro-Ed.

Higgins S: Motor skill acquisition, *Phys Ther* 71:123-139, 1991.

Kamhi AG: Dual perspectives on choosing treatment approaches to use or not to use: factors that influence the selection of new treatment approaches, *Lang Speech Hear Serv Sch* 30:92-97, 1999.

Kamhi AG: Summary, reflections, and future directions. In Kamhi AG, Pollock KE, editors: *Phonological disorders in children,* Baltimore, 2005, Paul H Brookes.

Kent RD, Lybolt JT: Techniques of therapy based in motor learning theory. In Perkins WH, editor: *Current therapy of communication disorders: general principles of therapy,* New York, 1982, Thieme-Stratton.

Kwiatkowski J, Shriberg LD: The capability-focus treatment framework for child speech disorders, *Am J Speech Lang Pathol* 7:27-38, 1998.

Ling D: *Speech and the hearing impaired child: theory and practice,* ed 2, Washington, DC, 2002, The Alexander Graham Bell Association for the Deaf and Hard of Hearing.

Munson B, Edwards J, Beckman ME: Phonological knowledge in typical and atypical speech-sound development, *Top Lang Disord* 25:190-206, 2005a.

Munson B, Edwards J, Beckman ME: Relationships between nonword repetition accuracy and other measures of linguistic development in children with phonological disorders, *J Speech Hear Res* 48:61-78, 2005b.

Olswang LB, Bain B: Data collection: monitoring children's treatment progress, *Am J Speech Lang Pathol* 3:55-66, 1994.

Paterson MM: Articulation and phonological disorders in hearing-impaired school-aged children with severe and profound sensorineural losses. In Bernthal J, Bankson N, editors: *Child phonology: characteristics, assessment, and intervention with special populations*, New York, 1994, Thieme Medical Publishers.

Peterson-Falzone SJ: Speech disorders related to craniofacial structural defects: I. In Lass NJ, McReynolds LV, Northern JL et al, editors: *Handbook of speech-language pathology and audiology*, Philadelphia, 1988, BC Decker.

Pipe P: *Practical programming*, New York, 1966, Holt, Rinehart, & Winston.

Rice ML, Hadley PA, Alexander AL: Social biases toward children with speech and language impairments: a correlative causal model of language limitations, *Appl Psycholinguist* 14:445-471, 1993.

Ruscello DM: Motor learning as a model for articulation instruction. In Costello JM, editor: *Speech disorders in children*, San Diego, 1984, College-Hill Press.

Ruscello DM: A motor skill learning treatment program for sound system disorders, *Semin Speech Lang* 14:106-118, 1993.

Ruscello DM: Residual phonological errors. In Kent R, editor: *The MIT Encyclopedia of communication disorders*, New York, 2003, Delmar Learning.

Rvachew S: The importance of phonetic factors in phonological intervention. In Kamhi AG, Pollock KE, editors: *Phonological disorders in children*, Baltimore, 2005, Paul H Brookes.

Schmidt RA, Wrisberg CA: *Motor learning and performance*, ed 2, Champaign, Ill, 2000, Human Kinetics.

Schwartz RG: Clinical applications of recent advances in phonological theory, *Lang Speech Hear Serv Sch* 23:269-276, 1992.

Shelton RL: Grand rounds for sound system disorder. Conclusion: what was learned, *Semin Speech Lang* 14:166-178, 1993.

Shelton RL, McReynolds LV: Functional articulation disorders: preliminaries to treatment. In Lass NJ, editor: *Speech and language: advances in basic research and practice*, New York, 1979, Academic Press.

Shriberg LD: Five subtypes of developmental phonological disorders, *Clin Commun Disord* 4:38-53, 1994.

Shriberg LD, Kwiatkowski J: Phonological disorders II: a conceptual framework for management, *J Speech Hear Disord* 47:242-256, 1982.

Shriberg LD, Kwiatkowski J: Developmental phonological disorders I: a clinical profile, *J Speech Hear Res* 37:1100-1126, 1994.

Skelton SL: Concurrent task sequencing in single-phoneme phonologic treatment and generalization, *J Commun Disord* 37:131-156, 2004.

St. Louis KO, Ruscello DM, Lundeen C: *Coexistence of communication disorders in schoolchildren,* ASHA Monograph 27, Rockville, Md, 1992, ASHA.

Tyler AA, Sandoval KT: Preschoolers with phonological and language disorders, *Lang Speech Hear Serv Sch* 25:215-234, 1994.

Weiss AL: The child as agent for change in therapy for phonological disorders, *Child Lang Teach Ther* 20:221-244, 2004.

Williams AL: The use of single-subject designs in clinical practice, *Clin Commun Disord* 3:47-58, 1993.

Williams AL: *Speech disorders resource guide for preschool children,* Clifton Park, NY, 2003, Singular.

Winitz H: *Articulatory acquisition and behavior,* New York, 1969, Appleton-Century-Crofts.

Yorkston KM, Beukelman DR, Strand EA et al: *Management of motor speech disorders in children and adults,* Austin, Tex, 1999, Pro-Ed.

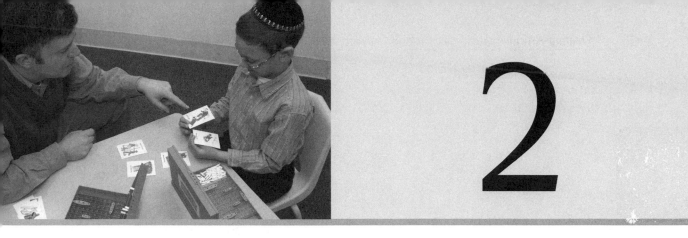

Sound System Treatment for Children with Functional Speech Sound Disorders

minimal pairs
multiple oppositions
multiple phoneme collapse
neighborhood density
nonmajor class features
oral motor treatment (OMT)
phoneme contrast
phonetic placement
phonotactic constraints
recasts
sonorant feature
speed drills
stop sounds
syllable structure
vowels
word frequency

LEARNING GOALS ■■■■
■ Outline the basic components
   involved in the restructuring of a
   child's sound system.

■ Summarize the following phonemic
   treatments: minimal pairs, multiple
   opposition, maximal opposition,
   morphosyntax, and conversational
   dialogues.
■ Summarize the following
   phonological processing
   approaches to treatment: metaphon
   and cycles.
■ Summarize the continuum of
   phonetic treatment activities, from
   isolation sound teaching through
   conversation.
■ Discuss the various phases and
   components of two "hybrid" treatment
   approaches: representation based and
   collaborative.
■ Identify some of the abiding issues
   that remain in the treatment of sound
   system disorders.

Treatments for sound system disorders are based on different theoretical perspectives. Chapter 1 discussed the theories that govern how clinicians treat clients and methodology to measure the response of clients to treatment. This chapter presents treatments that are currently used to remediate clients with sound system disorders. The literature frequently discusses treatments in terms of a dichotomy: On the one hand, a motor-learning approach (phonetic, traditional) is used; on the other hand, a linguistic approach (phonemic, cognitive-linguistic) is used. However, some treatment methods embody the features of both treatments. This chapter uses this dichotomy for organizational purposes, as well as to discuss treatment methods that embody features of both approaches.

Before the discussion of different treatments, drawing a distinction between motor-based and linguistic-based approaches to treatment is useful. In motor-based approaches, clinicians focus their attention on the phonetic or physical aspects of a sound and typically treat the sound system disorder on a sound-by-sound basis (Bauman-Waengler, 2004; Bernthal and Bankson, 2004; Lowe, 1994). The clinician provides opportunities for practice under the guise of motor skill learning to perfect sound production skills that he or she wishes to incorporate into the client's phonetic repertoire (Ruscello, 1993). The reader should note that in a motor-based approach, the clinician assumes that the child has the underlying representation or knowledge of the phoneme. That is, this knowledge is part of the child's phonological makeup, but the client has not learned the physical movements necessary to produce the sound or replaces the required movement pattern with another pattern. This is in contrast to the linguistic approach in which the underlying assumption is that the client has only partial or incomplete knowledge of the phonological system (Bernthal and Bankson, 2004). Practice is not the primary end of treatment; instead the clinician attempts to present the client with opportunities to restructure the phonological system.

In summary, motor-based approaches focus on developing the client's phonetic performance, whereas linguistic approaches focus on developing the client's phonological knowledge (Williams, 2003). Treatment data support both approaches (Gierut, 1998), but client, clinician, and caregiver factors influence which treatment is used for a specific client (see Chapter 1). The clinician has the ultimate responsibility for selecting, implementing, and evaluating the client's response to the treatment chosen. Additionally, clinicians must also be aware of two more qualifiers to this discussion. First, clear definitive distinctions between phonetic- and phonemic-based sound system disorders cannot always be established (Davis, 2005; Kahmi, 2005). Second, some clinicians have developed treatment approaches that incorporate both phonetic and phonemic features (Bowen and Cupples, 1999; Rvachew, 2005).

Motor-based treatment approaches focus on development of a client's phonetic performance, whereas linguistic treatment approaches focus on the development of a client's phonological knowledge.

Research Note

Williams, 2003.

Initially the clinician must carefully assess the child's sound system to determine whether a problem exists (Tyler, 2005a). Davis (2005) provides a cogent discussion of the assessment of sound system disorders and identifies important diagnostic issues that clinicians need to consider when engaged in this process. The diagnosis of a sound system disorder as the primary communication problem implies that treatment is necessary. The clinician will then treat the client using an intervention approach appropriate for the sound system disorder that was diagnosed (Figure 2-1).

Box 2-1 summarizes the process that is typically used. A comprehensive analysis of the child's sound system is first undertaken so that the disorder is identified. This involves conducting independent and relational analyses of the client's sound system disorder. This information and other relevant client, clinician, and caregiver factors are considered to select the appropriate treatment approach. After the approach has been determined, the clinician needs to formulate the appropriate terminal goal or goals for treatment. What is the goal of treatment for the time period of treatment? What is a realistic, achievable goal for the client? Baseline performance data of the client on treatment targets and (if appropriate) non–treatment control targets are collected before treatment. This is followed by the implementation of the treatment under either operant or motor skill principles of learning. During treatment, the clinician examines the client's performance by monitoring the response to training trials and probing for generalization. The collection of performance data allows the clinician to advance the client or alter treatment activities and determine whether the treatment is effective in advancing generalization.

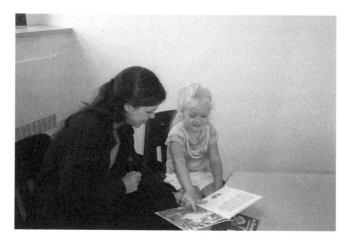

Figure **2-1** ■ Client undergoes treatment for a sound system disorder.

BOX 2-1 *Selecting and Implementing Treatment for a Sound System Disorder*

1. Carry out a comprehensive assessment of the client's sound system disorder.
   a. Independent analysis
   b. Relational analysis
2. Consider other relevant client, clinician, and caregiver factors.
3. Select the treatment approach appropriate for the client.
4. Develop appropriate terminal goals for the treatment period.
5. Create baseline goals to determine pretreatment levels of performance.
6. Implement the teaching approach.
   a. Introduce perception and production activities appropriate for the client.
   b. Establish response accuracy criteria to establish mastery of individual training activities.
7. Monitor the client's performance of the treatment.
   a. Collect daily performance data.
   b. Carry out periodic generalization assessments.

RESTRUCTURING THE CHILD'S SOUND SYSTEM

Phonemic Contrast

A linguistic approach to treatment may take a number of different forms, but the primary aim is to develop the phonemic distinctions of the ambient language (Barlow and Gierut, 2002). One of the earliest therapies was that of **minimal pairs** (Weiner, 1981), used initially from the viewpoint of phonological process analysis. However, this therapy has also been part of treatment based on feature analysis and productive phonological knowledge perspectives. Minimal pairs are words that differ by a single phoneme, thus signaling a meaning difference. The minimal pair /so-to/ illustrates two words, which have the same **vowel** but are different in reference to the prevocalic consonant and signal different lexical meaning. A traditional distinctive feature analysis of the consonants shows that they differ in terms of the manner of production; /s/ is a fricative and /t/ is a stop. The two phonemes also share features because they are both produced at the alveolar point of articulation and are voiceless. The minimal pair /so-go/ differs on all three feature dimensions; differences are seen in reference to voicing, place of articulation, and manner of articulation. A client may substitute or delete sounds and create **homonymy** (Bernthal and Bankson, 2004). That is, a collapse of phonemic contrast or contrasts occurs, and the collapse may have an effect on the client's intelligibility. For example, a client who uses /t/ in appropriate lexical contexts and also substitutes /t/ for /s/ may exhibit homonymy. The words *so-toe* are produced as *to-toe*. In attempting to restructure the client's sound system, the clinician uses minimal pairs to create meaning differences, thus fostering a restructuring.

Research Note	The primary aim of any form of linguistic treatment is to develop the phonemic distinctions of the ambient language.

Barlow and Gierut, 2002.

Variations of minimal-pairs treatment are also used to restructure a client's sound system (Gierut, 2005; Williams, 2003). These refinements in **phoneme contrast** are designed to increase the efficiency of intervention by facilitating widespread change in the child's phonemic system. Williams (2003) developed the multiple oppositions treatment, which addresses multiple-phoneme collapse, and Gierut (2005) and her research associates created maximal opposition. **Maximal opposition** is designed to confront clients with phonemic contrasts that differ according to major production class features.

Selecting Treatment Targets

Explicit in the linguistic approaches are also specific selection criteria for the development of treatment targets that are based on linguistic complexity (Gierut, 2001; Williams, 2003). That is, treatment directed to more complex linguistic properties is purported to result in greater system change for the client. The notion of using linguistic complexity differs from traditional phonetic approaches that use less complex selection metrics in their target selection criteria (Bernthal and Bankson, 2004). Traditional approaches generally target early-acquired sounds that are absent from the child's sound inventory and are stimulable, whereas linguistic approaches consider linguistic variables such as markedness, as well as lexical, phonetic, and phonemic complexity.

Some researchers believe that treatment directed to more complex linguistic properties results in greater system change for the client.

Research Note

Gierut, 2001; Williams, 2003.

Markedness

Proponents of phonemic approaches recommend teaching marked phonological features before unmarked features (Gierut, 2001; Williams, 2003). **Markedness** is a linguistic property of language. A marked feature in a language implies an unmarked feature. For example, voicing is a marked feature and implies an unmarked feature of voicelessness. That is, all languages have voiced sounds and, in most cases, voiced and voiceless sounds; however, no languages are composed of just voiceless sounds. Consequently, voicing is a marked feature. The following list contains some marked properties to consider in treatment selection:

- Treating voiced obstruent sounds may facilitate the acquisition of voiceless obstruent sounds.
- Treating **fricatives** may facilitate the acquisition of stops.
- Treating **affricates** may facilitate the acquisition of fricatives.
- Treating liquids may facilitate the acquisition of nasals.
- Treating clusters may facilitate the acquisition of singleton consonants.
- Treating later-developing clusters may facilitate the acquisition of early-developing clusters.

Lexical Complexity

Investigators have examined different properties of words that make up one's lexicon (Gierut, 2001). In particular, word frequency and neighborhood density have been the subject of study (Morrisette and Gierut, 2002). **Word frequency** is the regularity with which a particular word occurs in a language (Kucera and Francis, 1967), and studies indicate that subjects identify high-frequency words more readily than low-frequency words. **Neighborhood density** is a metric for the number of words that differ minimally in phonetic makeup from a specific word in terms of a single phoneme substitution, deletion, or addition. For example, the words *tea, stow,* and *doe* are neighbors of the word *toe* because they vary in terms of a single phoneme difference. Research findings indicate that words from low-density neighborhoods, which have limited phonetic linkages with other words, generally are easier to identify than high-density words.

Preliminary findings reported by Morrisette and Gierut for preschool children with severe sound system disorders indicate that using high-frequency words in treatment facilitates greater generalization than low-frequency words. However, no clear-cut generalization trend was found when using either high-density or low-density words. The data suggest that clinicians consider using high-frequency words in the treatment paradigm.

Research Note	Preliminary studies indicate that individuals identify high-frequency words more readily than low-frequency words. Data also indicate that more extensive generalization may be associated with the use of high-frequency words.

Morrissette and Gierut, 2002.

Phonetic and Phonemic Complexity

Gierut (2001) summarized a number of research investigations that studied different phonetic and phonemic factors in treatment. The overall findings suggest that the clinician should account for the following when treating phonemic targets:
- Treat sounds that are not stimulable.
- Treat sounds that are acoustically undifferentiated.
- Treat sounds that are absent from the child's inventory of sounds.
- Treat sounds that are developmentally later acquired rather than earlier acquired sounds.

PHONEMIC TREATMENT

Minimal Pairs

A training plan for a client using minimal pairs consists of several steps designed to establish the phonemic contrast through perception and production activities. The steps used to implement this treatment are outlined in the following sections (Box 2-2).

Step 1: Perception

Select four to eight sets of minimal pairs that can be displayed via pictures. If it is difficult to generate a sufficient number of pictures, then nonce items may be used. Meaning may be introduced by associating a pictorial shape with the nonce item (see Chapter 1). For discussion, assume that the child is using /t/ in substitution of /s/ and the minimal

---

> **BOX 2-2** *Summary of Steps in Minimal-Pairs Treatment*
>
> **Step 1: Perception (Optional)**
> Clinician selects and presents pictures to the client, providing stimulus cues for items to be used in treatment.
>
> **Step 2: Phonetic Production (Optional)**
> Clinician probes the client's phonetic-production skills and teaches placement of target sound, if necessary.
>
> **Step 3: Minimal Pairs**
> Clinician presents minimal pairs individually and asks the client to produce each item.
>
> **Step 4: Minimal Pairs in Context**
> Clinician incorporates minimal pairs in contextual practice material, often within stereotypical carrier sentences.

---

pairs selected are *two-sue, toe-sew, tea-sea, tap-sap,* and *tip-sip.* The pictures of each are introduced to the child and named by the clinician before introducing the perceptual task so that the child is familiar with the treatment items. The client would then be engaged in the perceptual task. The clinician displays the pictures and provides stimulus cues (e.g., "I want you to show me the picture that I say. Show me sea."). The client's response is to identify the correct item. This is an optional step that may or may not be included in treatment. In some applications of minimal pairs, an introductory perceptual step is not part of the minimal-pairs treatment (Weiner, 1981).

Some authors also use imagery to create distinctions between minimal pairs. Klein (1996) describes imagery as a cognitive process that is used to develop a phonological contrast through the use of semantic anchors or descriptions. Descriptive terms are used to label the feature contrast undergoing treatment. In the previous example of a stop being used in place of a fricative, the distinction between *sounds that are long sounding* and *sounds that are short sounding* might be introduced. The fricative would be the long-sounding sound and initially presented in a slightly prolonged manner within the target words. The **stop sound,** or short-sounding sound, could be portrayed as a very quickly articulated sound as produced in words. Imagery is also used in other phonemic approaches (discussed later in the chapter).

Step 2: Phonetic Production

Step 2 is also optional; however, some clinicians use it when the client does not have the phonetic skills to produce the target sound. Bernthal and Bankson (2004) recommend that the clinician probe the client's phonetic-production skills and teach placement of the target sound, if necessary, so that the client has imitative control of the target sound in words. Tyler and colleagues (1987) also provide a word imitation step, with words containing the target sound. The client must demonstrate imitative control of the target in words before advancing to actual minimal-pairs contrast. Some authors do not include phonetic practice as a precursor to the introduction of minimal pairs (Weiner, 1981). For example, Klein (1996) indicates that minimal pairs are designed to present the client with phonemic contrasts; consequently, phonetic teaching procedures such as placement instructions and imitative cues are not part of a "pure" linguistic teaching approach.

Step 3: Minimal Pairs

The minimal pairs are presented individually, and the client is instructed to produce each of the items. For example, the clinician presents pictures of the minimal pair /tea-sea/ (Figure 2-2) and instructs the client to identify spontaneously each picture (e.g., "I want you to name the picture that I point to. Ready, name this picture." Tyler (2005b) describes a variation wherein the clinician plays "Go Fish" with the client. The clinician has pictures of the minimal pairs, and the client is given only pictures of the target words. The client is instructed to produce the target words to receive the picture match from the clinician. If the client errs in production, then the picture representing the minimal-pairs contrast will be given to the client, rather than the target word to create a communication mismatch. This places the client in a communication interaction that is unsuccessful and can facilitate the development of the appropriate phonemic contrast. A number of different ways can be used to present the minimal pairs and elicit the responses spontaneously.

At this level of treatment the clinician must have an operational definition of a correct response. Some authors provide the client with positive feedback for the elimination of the error, not the specific target sound (Saben and Ingham, 1991), whereas others define the response as the specific phoneme (Tyler et al., 1987). For instance, a client may delete fricatives in the postvocalic position and the minimal pair /my-mice/ may be used. If the child's response to /mice/ contained a postvocalic fricative other than /s/, then positive affirmation would be given because the client is learning the rule. However, this aspect of minimal-pairs treatment remains controversial. Tyler (2005b) indicates that the client should have imitative control of the target in some words before using minimal pairs. If not, then the minimal-pairs activity may be frus-

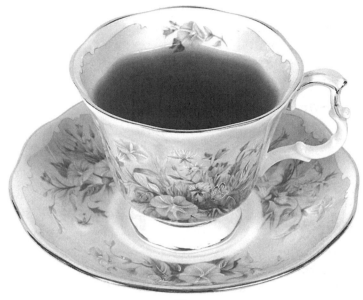

Tea

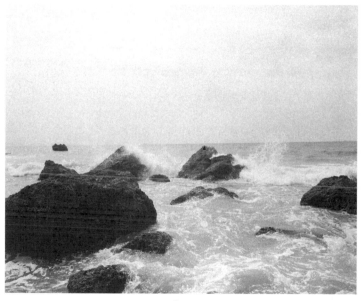

Sea

Figure 2-2 ■ Examples of pictures that may be used as part of the minimal-pairs treatment. (Copyright 2007, JupiterImages Corporation.)

trating because the client does not meet with success. Clinicians must be cognizant of this issue when introducing the actual production of minimal pairs and determine the most beneficial option for the client. It may be necessary to include an imitative phonetic step before having the client produce the pairs spontaneously.

Step 4: Minimal Pairs in Context

The final step is to incorporate the minimal pairs in contextual practice material. This is generally accomplished by incorporating the pairs in stereotypical **carrier sentences** (e.g., "I see a ___ and a ___"). When the client achieves the predetermined response accuracy criterion, practice may shift to individual use of the targets in carrier sentences (e.g., "I am pointing to the ___"). The clinician may find that other activities may need to be introduced (e.g., conversational practice), but the breadth of activity will depend in large part on the generalization of the client. As discussed in Chapter 1, measurement of generalization is critical to evaluating the success of the treatment and determining whether certain treatment activities are needed.

CASE STUDY 2-1

Minimal Pairs: A Phonemic Approach to Treatment

D.B. is a 4-year, 6-month-old boy who was seen for an assessment at the referral of his family physician. The physician and D.B.'s family had concerns regarding delayed speech development and problems with being understood by others. The child attended a preschool program for the past 2 years, and his mother indicated that he is not as easy to understand as his peers. She stated that he deletes some sounds, particularly at the end of words, and substitutes some sounds for other sounds. His mother also reported that she has two older children, but they did not experience any problems with speech and language development. An analysis of the client's sound system indicated a consonant inventory of /p, b, t, d/, /θ, ð, h/, /w, j, l/, /m, n, ŋ/ and all vowels and diphthongs. The most prominent errors were the use of the stops /t, d/ in place of the alveolar and palatal fricatives and affricates in the prevocalic and intervocalic positions, as well as the deletion of obstruent sounds in the postvocalic position. The client was stimulable for /k, g/. The client used V, CV, VC, and CVC syllable shapes. Intelligibility was judged to be in the moderate to severe range because of inventory constraints and positional constraints affecting obstruents. Hearing testing indicated that acuity was normal bilaterally. An oral examination was unremarkable. Language testing revealed a mild receptive delay and a moderate delay in expressive language.

The child was enrolled for 24 treatment sessions, which were 1 hour in duration. A phonemic approach to treatment was used because of the pattern of sound system errors displayed. Minimal pairs were used to target the two major sound system errors that involved the substitution of alveolar stops for lingual fricatives and affricates and the deletion of obstruents in the final position. The phoneme /z/ was selected as the target for the alveolar stop substitution because it was not stimulable and was a later developing sound. It was also chosen because voiced obstruents may facilitate the development of voiceless obstruents (see text discussion). The phoneme /v/ was chosen as the postvocalic target because of the same selection criteria. Word pairs such as *zoo-due, zip-dip, zee-dee,* and *zoom-doom* were used to contrast the alveolar stop substitution, and word pairs *moo-move, way-wave, lee-leave,* and *dry-drive* were used to contrast the postvocalic positional constraint.

The initial step of the treatment was to introduce the minimal pairs. Pictures of the minimal pairs were presented to the client, and the items were produced for the client. After the introduction, the items were presented individually and the client was asked to identify each. This was followed by production of the pairs by the client. Each pair was presented, and the client was to produce the pairs spontaneously. Because D.B. did not have the phonetic skills requisite to production of the minimal-pair targets /z, v/, an intermediate phonetic teaching step was included. D.B. was taught phonetic placement of /z, v/ in isolation and imitative production of the minimal pairs before spontaneous practice. The final step was incorporation of the minimal pairs in contextual practice material. The clinician did this by incorporating the pairs in stereotypical carrier sentences (e.g., "I see a ____ and a ____"). Probe measures taken periodically during treatment and posttreatment showed improvement from baseline levels of response. Response generalization for both /z/ and /v/ were identified at the word level, and the targeted sounds also began to emerge in spontaneous conversation. Generalization of untaught sounds /f/, /s/, and /ʃ/ was found at the spontaneous word level.

Commentary

D.B. had a moderately severe problem that has improved with treatment. Generalization of targets and related sounds indicate that the treatment was an effective agent for sound system change. His profile is one of a child with coexisting language and phonology issues. The treatment allowed the client to begin restructuring his sound system through minimal contrast. The minimal-pair contrast, along with language therapy, will continue so that additional gains in phonology and language may be realized.

Multiple Oppositions

Williams (2003, 2005, 2006) has conducted substantive treatment research and studied clients with severe phonological disorders. Some of the clients demonstrated **multiple phoneme collapse** (i.e., one phoneme is used in place of many phonemes). Rather than target a single contrast as in minimal pairs, Williams reasoned that it would be more beneficial to target multiple-phoneme collapse through treatment designated as **multiple oppositions**. That is, because a general rule is operating, therapy must be directed to the rule and not subsets of the rule. For example, a client who uses /t/ for /t/, /s/, /k/, and /ʃ/ would benefit from an integrated treatment of the phoneme collapse rather than individual minimal-pair sets. Multiple opposition sets such as *two-sue, two-coo, two-shoe* would be used to address multiple errors that stem from a single rule. The client is exposed to the gestalt so that he or she may reorganize the phonological system in a structured, systematic, and efficient manner. The phases of this treatment approach are outlined in the following sections (Box 2-3).

Phase 1: Introduction

The initial or introductory part of the treatment contains three components. The first component is designed to present the rule that is being taught, the second is to introduce the vocabulary to be used, and the third is production of the sound contrasts, as follows:

1. The first step in this treatment is presentation of the phonological rule by contrasting what the child does with what he or she needs to do. Because the contrast may be abstract for the child, the clinician needs to structure this activity at the child's level. The idea is to present the rule in a concrete manner. One way of achieving this goal is to use imagery (as discussed under Minimal Pairs). For example, a child needing to develop the continuant feature in place of the stop feature might be exposed to the "pouring sound" versus the "dripping sound." The clinician could contrast a *spigot with pouring water* to introduce the fricative with a *spigot of dripping water*, which represents the stop feature. Place-feature errors could be anchored for the child by drawing a distinction between *sounds made in the front of the mouth* and *sounds made in the back of the mouth*. Sound deletions associated with final consonants might be presented as "whole words" versus part words. A visual anchor of small blocks representing each sound could be contrasted with a missing block to signal the missing sound. No completion criteria exist for this step. Williams (2003) indicates

---

BOX 2-3 *Summary of Phases in Multiple-Oppositions Treatment*

Phase 1

Clinician presents phonological rule by contrasting what the client does with what he or she should do.

Clinician introduces vocabulary.

Clinician provides an imitative model of the contrastive pairs along with the pictorial references, and he or she asks the client to produce the word pairs.

Phase 2

Clinician produces pictures of the word pairs, and the client practices them under imitative and spontaneous conditions. Clients should produce 60 to 100 responses per 30-minute session.

Interactive play is also incorporated into this phase.

Phase 3

Client has achieved spontaneous production of the contrasts, and practice shifts to activities that promote spontaneous use through various games and techniques.

Data from Williams AL: *Speech disorders resource guide for preschool children*, Clifton Park, NJ, 2003, Thomson Delmar Learning; Williams AL: A model and structure for phonological intervention. In Kamhi AG, Pollock KE, editors: *Phonological disorders in children*, Baltimore, 2005, Paul H Brookes Publishing, pp 189-199; Williams AL: *Sound contrasts in phonology (SCIP)*, Eau Claire, Wis, 2006, Thinking Publications (CD-ROM).

that the child must be involved actively in this step to make certain that he or she understands the concept (phonological rule). Williams estimates that the activity should require approximately 15 to 20 minutes.

2. The next step is introduction of vocabulary so that the child becomes familiar with the pictures that represent the desired treatment pairs. This is an identification phase for the client so that he or she is totally familiar with the practice stimuli. Williams (2003) recommends that each picture be displayed and the clinician produce each item. The author believes that is also helpful to tell a short story about each item to assist the child in associating the picture with the desired vocabulary items.

3. The final part of the introductory phase is actual production of the stimuli imitatively. The clinician provides an imitative model of the contrastive pairs *tea-sea*, while also providing the pictorial references. The child is required to produce the word pairs. Linguistic feedback

is provided to the child concerning the accuracy of the productions. For example, if the previous pair was produced as *tea-tea*, then the clinician might say, "We drink tea (pointing to the picture of tea), but the boat floats in the sea (pointing to the picture of the sea)." Williams (2003) cautions that in some cases, the clinician may need to break down the pairs and practice the words separately. After the child can produce the stimuli separately, the contrastive word pairs are reintroduced.

Research Note	In step 2, it may be helpful to tell a story about the picture to help the client associate that image with the desired vocabulary item.

Williams, 2003.

No accuracy criteria exist that the client must meet for any of the three steps. The purpose of the introductory phase is to (1) develop an awareness of the rule that is being taught, (2) present the paired treatment items that contain the treatment contrasts, and (3) elicit imitative production of the treatment pairs. The primary goal is to build a foundation for the phases that follow.

Phase 2: Production

Phase 2 is a production phase designed to elicit imitative responses of the contrasts and then shift to spontaneous production. Interactive-play situations that focus on the target contrasts are also incorporated into this phase. Williams (2003) stresses the need for the child to concentrate on the contrasts and not be distracted from the treatment through the use of board games. The author recommends that clients should produce between 60 and 100 responses per 30-minute session. This is a time for clinical focus on the part of the child. Moreover, this phase of treatment frequently takes the most time because the client is developing the contrasts.

Research Note	In phase 2, clients should practice the target words frequently in treatment sessions.

Williams, 2003.

In a typical practice session, the clinician introduces pictures of the word pairs and then they are practiced. As the child begins to produce the contrastive pairs, the clinician varies the order of the pairs to stress the salience of the contrasts and minimize simple articulatory repetition. For instance, the pair *tip-sip* would also be presented as *sip-tip*. The pairs are practiced under both imitative and spontaneous conditions. First, the child practices the pairs via imitation until a criterion of 70% accuracy has been achieved for two consecutive training sets. A training set is a block of responses that are used to measure the client's response to the treatment. If the client were practicing four multiple-opposition contrasts *tip-kip, tip-sip, tip-ship, tip-chip*, and each pair was presented five times, then a total of 20 presentations would exist in a training set. The client would need to achieve 70% accuracy (at least 14 of the contrasts would need to be judged correct) in each of two consecutive training sets to shift from imitative to spontaneous practice. The spontaneous practice is completed when the child achieves an accuracy criterion of 90% across two consecutive training sets. The author indicates that a training set consists of 20 to 50 responses; the number of responses depends on the number of contrasts being taught.

In addition to the contrastive word practice, interactive play with the targets is carried out after practice of the contrasts. Interactive play is used to provide a more naturalistic context for practice of the targets. That is, the play is designed to simulate actual conditions wherein the client needs to use the target contrasts appropriately. Williams (2003) explains that the child needs opportunities to help develop the new phonological rule and also use the target contrasts in more naturalistic contexts. The clinician should use an activity that enables him or her to model treatment targets and furnish opportunities for the client to produce the practice targets in words. For example, the clinician might read a book to the child and stress the production of words that contain the target words. The child would be prompted to produce some of those targets, which have been introduced in treatment. Other clinician-directed activities such as interactive play (e.g., artwork, pretend play) might be used to create other conversational conditions.

Interactive play provides the client with needed opportunities to help him or her develop the new phonological rule and use the target contrasts in more naturalistic contexts.

Research Note

Williams, 2003.

Phase 3: Spontaneous Use

At phase 3 the child has achieved spontaneous production of the contrasts; consequently, practice shifts to activities that promote spontaneous use. Using the paired contrasts is no longer necessary because the new treatment activities provide contexts for use of the newly acquired phonological targets. The aim is to provide different opportunities in more naturalistic contexts that are typically appealing for young clients. For example, the child and the clinician may take turns and engage in games such as matching contrastive pairs (Go Fish, concentration), or the child "instructs" the clinician to point to different pictures that he or she identifies. Feedback is an important component that is continually provided so that the client is made aware of correct and incorrect productions.

No response completion criterion exists for phase 3 practice activities as used in phase 2; instead, completion is based on response generalization data that have been collected throughout treatment (see Chapter 1 for further information). Williams (2003) recommends that generalization probes of 10 words for each target sound in the position treated be constructed and administered at every third session to assess response generalization. If the child achieves an accuracy level of 90% on a generalization probe, then phase 3 is completed. A conversational probe to assess use of the contrasts in spontaneous speech follows the achievement of the generalization criterion. Using criteria advocated by Fey (1986), therapy is concluded for the treatment opposition if the client achieves 50% accuracy or higher in spontaneous speech for the phonological contrasts being taught.

Research Note	Generalization probes of 10 words for each target sound in the position treated should be constructed and administered at every third treatment session to assess response generalization.

Williams, 2003.

Phase 4: Conversation

Phase 4 is used for clients who are not generalizing the target sounds to spontaneous conversation. The clinician engages the child in conversation and uses **recasts** of the child's error productions as adapted from the work of Camarata (1993). The recasts are immediate and contingent on the error productions of the child as monitored through conversational interchanges, but they are not to distract from the spontaneity of the conversational interchange. The linguistic feedback furnished to the client is a correct model provided immediately after an incorrect production and a positive verbal affirmation for correct productions. For example, the client might say "I want a potato *tip*." The clinician saying, "Yes, a potato *chip*," would follow that. In the example, the clinician's response immediately follows the error; however, it does not detract from the conversational interchange. Similarly, a response such as "I put a <u>c</u>heck mark on it" would be followed by the clinician's "Yes, you are correct." No direct requests are given for imitation during conversational sessions. The clinician must use activities and materials that allow for numerous response opportunities. Response generalization probes of words continue during this phase, with the goal of achieving the 90% criterion. Achievement of the criterion would be followed by a conversational probe and termination of the treatment opposition if the 50% spontaneous conversational probe criterion was met.

CASE STUDY 2-2

Multiple Oppositions: A Phonemic Approach to Treatment

T.S. is a 4-year-old girl who was referred for an assessment because her mother was concerned about the child's lack of speech development and inability to be understood. The girl had undergone an earlier evaluation at another facility and was given a provisional diagnosis of childhood apraxia of speech (CAS). According to the child's mother, T.S. talked very little, and what few words she did say were unintelligible. Her primary mode of communication was through idiosyncratic signing and gestures, and she became frustrated and upset when she was not understood. All other developmental milestones in terms of cognitive, motor, and social skills were reported to be within the normal limits. T.S. lives at home with her mother, father, older brother, and younger sister. For approximately 3 months at the other facility, treatment was conducted using a phonetic approach, with goals consisting of imitating and spontaneously producing single-word utterances. T.S. was seen for 12 sessions; each was 60 minutes in length. A clinical summary indicated that very little progress was made, and the child remained unintelligible.

An analysis of the client's sound system patterns revealed a consonant inventory of /b/, /m/, /h/ and the vowels /i, I, e, u, a, æ/. Deletion errors were the predominant type of problem identified; inventory constraint was the major problem identified during testing. With the exception of

/b/, all obstruents were missing from the client's inventory, as were liquids and glides. The /m/ was the only nasal present. Hypernasality was identified as a feature during the production of vowels. Syllabic structure consisted of the simple syllable shapes V and CV; she also used the vowel configuration V-V in place of multisyllabic words. T.S. was stimulable for /f/, /v/, /j/, and /w/. The oral mechanism was unremarkable, and pure tone thresholds were within normal limits. Language testing indicated normal receptive language skills and a delay of approximately 1 year in expressive language skills.

Sound system treatment for T.S. at the author's facility was changed because of her lack of progress and the fact that clinicians felt she did not meet the diagnostic criteria for CAS. Because the child exhibited extensive phoneme collapse, it was decided that a phonemic approach to therapy would be used. The multiple-oppositions approach (Williams, 2003) was selected to treat T.S.'s phonological impairment. Rather than target a single contrast as used with minimal pairs, the clinicians felt that treatment would be more beneficial by targeting the multiple-phoneme collapse. Using the selection criteria of markedness and phonetic and phonemic complexity for phonological treatment (see text discussion), the alveolar voiced fricative /z/ was chosen, along with the palatal voiceless fricative /ʃ/ and the alveolar liquid /l/. The targets were selected because voiced obstruents may facilitate the acquisition of voiceless obstruents (/z/), targeting fricatives may facilitate the acquisition of stops (/z, ʃ/), and sounds that are not stimulable are taught before sounds that are stimulable (/z, ʃ, l/). Multiple-opposition sets such as *e-zee, e-she,* and *e-lee* were used to address the multiple errors that may stem from a single underlying phonological rule. The rationale was to expand the client's inventory and increase the use of CV syllable shapes. When T.S. completed the multiple-oppositions treatment for the 24 allotted sessions of 50 minutes per session, probe measures and posttreatment generalization measures of spontaneous word production and conversation showed gains in the consonant inventory and improved intelligibility. Response generalization for /p/, /v/, /t/, and /tʃ/ were found at the word level in addition to the selected treatment phonemes. The targeted sounds also began to emerge in spontaneous conversation. She began to use consistently CV shapes with the appearance of VC and CVCV combinations. Hypernasality was no longer perceived during the production of vowel sounds.

Commentary

Because only minimal progress was noted, use of phonetic treatment was discontinued. In-depth assessment was necessary to identify the client's sound system disorder and to make recommendations for future treatment. T.S. required a treatment that assisted her in developing phonological rules, not movements requisite to correct phonetic productions. The rapid change in the child's phonological system supported the use of the multiple-oppositions treatment. Treatment continued with the goal of further increasing T.S's sound inventory and phonotactics to include CVC shapes. In addition to the sound system treatment, expressive language therapy was carried out and needs to be continued.

Maximal Oppositions

Gierut (2005) proposes that the purpose of phonemic treatment is to expand the client's underlying knowledge of the ambient sound system. To this end, she suggests that *what* the clinician teaches a client is more critical than *how* the clinician teaches the client. Her research has centered on examining what is taught from the perspective of linguistic complexity. That is, more complex linguistic input to the client results in more extensive change in the client's sound system (Gierut, 1989, 1990). The author and her associates have conducted a number of single-subject, multiple-baseline studies and found that different generalization patterns emerge as a function of minimal-pair variations.

What the clinician teaches the client is more critical than how the clinician teaches. That is, more complex linguistic input results in more extensive change in the client's sound system.

Research Note

Gierut, 1989, 1990, 2005.

The minimal-pair alternations proposed by Barlow and Gierut (2002) pair phonemes that differ maximally in terms of their features, not minimally as with the original minimal-pairs treatment (discussed previously). A brief discussion of features is included so that the reader may follow the discussion. The features of voice, place, and manner are known as **nonmajor class features** and are used to delineate the features of sounds. The sound pair /s, t/ differs in terms of the manner of articulation and constitutes a minimal variation. Major class features distinguish the main sound categories of a language. They are typically the most prominent in languages and generally are some of the first features to appear during the child's acquisition of language. **Major**

class differences include vowels versus consonants, consonants versus glides, and sonorants versus obstruents, with the **feature contrasts** being syllabic, consonantal, and sonorant (Sloat et al., 1978). Syllabic sounds are produced with the greatest energy or prominence in a syllable. Vowels are syllabic sounds. The consonantal feature implies some constriction or complete blockage of the vocal tract. Sound classes sharing the consonantal feature are stops, fricatives, affricates, liquids, and nasals. Sounds with the **sonorant feature** are produced with a vocal tract shape that does not restrict sound energy from passing through either the oral or nasal cavities. Liquids, nasals, vowels, and glides share the sonorant feature. Table 2-1 categorizes the major class features.

With maximal oppositions, the clinician can manipulate major and nonmajor features to develop treatment pairs that will help the client expand his or her phonemic inventory (Barlow and Gierut, 2002). Accordingly, the clinician can pair a sound that is missing from the client's inventory with a sound that is functional in the child's inventory (or pair sounds that are both missing from the child's inventory). The preferred maximal opposition would be the selection of two sounds that are missing from the client's inventory and differ in terms of major class features. For example, if both /s/ and /w/ were missing from the child's inventory, then their pairing would create a maximal opposition that is a major class distinction *(see-we)*. The major class difference is consonantal /s/ versus sonorant /w/, and one would predict the most

Table 2-1
Summary of Major Class Features

SOUND CLASSES	SYLLABIC	CONSONANTAL	SONORANT
Liquids and nasals /r, l, m, n, ŋ/	–	+	+
Vowels	+	–	+
Glides /w, j/	–	–	+
Obstruents /p, b, t, d, k, g, tʃ, dʒ/ and /f, v, θ, ð, s, z, ʃ, ʒ/	–	+	–

+, Feature of the sound class; –, not a feature of the sound class.

substantial generalization. The clinician's development of maximal oppositions depends on the child's phonetic and phonemic inventories. Figure 2-3 presents a hierarchy of potential maximal oppositions for consideration. They are ordered from the least-predicted system-wide change to the most-predicted system-wide change.

The clinician should keep in mind that the maximal oppositions approach is predicated on the *what* to teach (Gierut, 2005). A clinician must carefully select targets based on the complexity metrics (see previous discussion of target selection criteria) and the different maximal opposition pairs. The actual treatment steps to be summarized (Box 2-4) are used for experimental purposes in a treatment research project known as the *Learnability Project* (www.indiana.edu/~sndlrng). The clinician needs to be cognizant of this and implement the treatment accordingly.

Step 1: Selecting Treatment Targets

After a comprehensive phonological assessment (Elbert and Gierut, 1986), the clinician applies the complexity metrics (discussed previously) to select targets for treatment. Initially those sounds that are missing from the child's inventory are selected for consideration as possible targets. After the pool has been established, sounds that are predicted to generalize from the treatment of another sound are eliminated. For example, the teaching of affricates predicts the development of fricatives. Additional considerations include sound stimulability and early

Least

Maximal Opposition Pairs

1. A new phoneme paired with a functional phoneme.
A nonmajor feature difference.

2a. Two new paired phonemes.
A nonmajor feature difference.

2b. A new phoneme paired with a functional phoneme.
A major feature difference.

3. Two new paired phonemes.
A major feature difference.

Most

Figure **2-3** ■ Ordering of maximal oppositions according to the amount and predicted change (from least to most). (Modified from Barlow JA, Gierut JA: Minimal pair approaches to phonological remediation, *Semin Speech Lang* 23:57-67, 2002.)

BOX 2-4   *Summary of Steps in Maximal-Opposition Treatment*

Step 1: Selection of Treatment Targets
Clinician conducts a comprehensive phonological analysis and applies the complexity metrics to select targets for treatment.

Step 2: Phonetic Production
Clinician instructs the client to imitate the target sound and accompanies each item with pictorial referents.

Step 3: Spontaneous Production
When the client achieves imitative control of the target sound or sounds, the clinician provides the pictorial representations and encourages the client to spontaneously reproduce them.

---

acquired sounds versus late sounds. In summary, an ideal maximal-opposition pair would be sounds that are missing from the sound inventory, are marked when compared with other sounds or sound classes, are not stimulable, and are later acquired. Sounds that are not selected for treatment are also sampled during baseline (and periodically during treatment) to monitor change in both treated and untreated sounds.

Step 2: Phonetic Production

The first production step consists of an imitative phase of production. The client is instructed to imitate the target sound as incorporated in the prevocalic position of words or nonce words. The items are accompanied by pictorial referents. Because this is an experimental treatment paradigm, the actual treatment step will vary depending on the research question. In some cases, imitative trials are with single words; in others, word pairs are used. Additionally, the use of words or nonce words as imitative stimuli will vary as a function of the research, and training stimuli are limited to between 6 and 16 items. Treatment of the sound in isolation is not used, but successive approximations of the target in context and placement cues are used when needed.

The imitative phase is carried out in a drill/play format (see Chapter 1), and clients are given response accuracy information after each training trial. Positive verbal cues are provided, contingent on each correct response. If the child produces an incorrect response, then the clinician provides feedback regarding correct placement of the target. This is followed by an imitative recue of the error and another production attempt by the client. A correct response of the recue is followed by positive verbal feedback. A second error response to the recue is ignored, and the next training item is presented to the client. Treatment at the imitative level is limited to a total of seven sessions or until the child achieves a response accuracy level of 75% for two consecutive training sessions, whichever is achieved first.

Step 3: Spontaneous Production

When the client achieves imitative control of the target or targets, treatment shifts to spontaneous production. The client is given the pictorial representations and spontaneously produces the items. The drill/play format is maintained, as is feedback regarding correct and incorrect responses. Achievement criteria for this step is the completion of 12 practice sessions or 90% response accuracy across three consecutive practice sessions, whichever is achieved first.

The treatment regimen ends at the spontaneous word level. Again, the reader should note that this treatment is used for experimental purposes. If clinicians use the treatment paradigm, then they may need to develop other activities to expand further the client's phonemic inventory. Generalization testing is also an important adjunct because it provides information on the degree of system-wide change and modifications that need to be introduced in treatment.

Other Linguistic-Based Approaches

Substantial numbers of clients have sound system disorders and coexisting problems in other aspects of language such as morphology and syntax (Tyler, 2002). Although the exact relationship among structural, semantic, and pragmatic components of language is unknown, interactions with phonology cannot be ignored. It follows that phonology is not independent from other components of language, and treatment should be directed not only to phonology but also to other components that are at variance with developmental expectations. The reader should note that approaches to be discussed focus on the totality of the language problem, not sound system errors specifically. These approaches are not to be confused with naturalistic elicitation techniques that focus on sound system errors such as conversational recasting, a treatment technique developed by Camarata (1993) and discussed previously. In her cogent discussion of language-based treatment, Tyler (2002) indicates that such an approach may be suitable for clients with language disorders that include sound system errors produced on a variable basis. That is, clients who are inconsistent in their production of sound system targets may be candidates for a language-based approach. Implicit with such a treatment approach is that interactions among the language domains will occur, and therapy for a language domain such as morphology will have a positive influence on the client's sound system errors (i.e., a top-down effect may occur).

Research Note	Clients with language disorders that include sound system errors produced inconsistently may be good candidates for language-based approaches to treatment.

Tyler, 2002.

Language-Based Treatment: Morphosyntax

An example of such a language-based treatment is that formulated by Tyler and colleagues (2002). The following three components are included in treatment:
1. Auditory awareness of linguistic targets
2. Focused stimulation
3. Elicited production of language targets

   Auditory awareness is used to enhance the client's consciousness of the language targets that are being introduced, whereas the focused-stimulation technique provides numerous examples of language targets in natural communicative contexts. Finally, elicitation tasks are used to facilitate practice of the language structure or structures. The different activities used for each component are based on different topics such as animals, community helpers, different events, and other such themes that may be of interest to the client. All three components are carried out in a treatment session, and accuracy performance criteria are not set but rather used to introduce a new language structure at each session. The treatment is a session-by-session immersion of a specific goal. Written scripts are prepared to guide the clinician in the conduct of treatment. Box 2-5 summarizes the morphosyntax treatment components.

Research Note	Components of morphosyntax treatment include the following:
	    1. Auditory awareness of linguistic targets
	    2. Focused stimulation
	    3. Elicited production of language targets

Tyler et al., 2002.

BOX 2-5 *Summary of Components in Morphosyntax Treatment*

Component 1: Auditory Awareness
Clinician uses books and songs to create an awareness of the language target.

Component 2: Focused Stimulation
Clinician presents the client with numerous examples of the language target in appropriate and functional contexts but does not prompt the client to respond.

Component 3: Elicited Production of Language Targets
Clinician uses a continuum of high-level to low-level structured-elicitation models to encourage the client to produce the target.

Data from Tyler AA, Lewis KE, Haskill A et al: Efficacy and cross domain effects of morphosyntax and phonology intervention, *Lang Speech Hear Serv Sch* 33:52-66, 2002.

Component 1: Auditory Awareness. Books and songs are used to create an awareness of the language target. For example, if the clinician were introducing regular comparative adjective forms (i.e., *-er*), then a book, a song, or both would be chosen that contains examples of the intended target such as, "The dog is *bigger* than the cat," with emphasis on the comparative form. Other examples would also be introduced so that the child is exposed to numerous examples of the language target.

Component 2: Focused Stimulation. The clinician presents the client with numerous examples of the language target in appropriate and functional contexts (Fey, 1986). The child is not prompted to respond, but the clinician attempts to structure the stimulation in a way that promotes the child's production of the language target. In the context of a focused-stimulation vignette, different elicitation techniques such as expansions, expatiations recasting, and false assertions are used.

Clinician: "My dog is bigger than yours." (Looking at pictures together, the clinician makes a false assertion about the size of the dogs.)

Client: "My doggie bigger."

Clinician: "Yes, your doggie is bigger." (Expansion used to add additional linguistic information.)

Client: "Yeah."

Clinician: "Are you sure your doggie is bigger?" (Sentence is recast in question form for the client.)

Client: "Yes, my doggie is bigger."

Component 3: Elicited Production of Language Targets. Component 3 involves the production of the target in structured-elicitation models that range from high- to low-level clinician prompting (Box 2-6). As the child acquires a language structure, clinician support can be altered from high to low support. High support consists of a forced-choice model that obligates the client to use the desired target (e.g., "Is this man in the picture taller or shorter than the other one?"). The reader should note that alternative choices are used to obligate the use of a specific language target. The cloze procedure is an intermediate-support technique in which the client is provided with information and must complete the request for the missing language structure (e.g., "This cow is big, but this cow is ___"). In this example the client must make a choice, but the choice involves the generation of a specific language response.

The final elicitation model is that of preparatory sets (Paul, 2007). This type of intervention activity is designed to heighten the client's awareness of the treatment goal and prepare the client for use of the target in different contexts. The client has been exposed through the three treatment components to the specific language goal with the idea of transfer to more naturalistic settings. The clinician demonstrates the target indirectly so that the client uses it in a more natural, communicative interaction. For instance, the clinician might provide a number of examples of the target and have the child produce the targets in sentence-level responses:

Clinician: "Billy, look at the book. This dog is bigger than that dog. Look over here. The boy is taller than his brother. Look at this. These girls are all bigger than their sister. Now, you take your book and tell me a little story. What is happening?"

Client: "That cow is bigger than the calf, and the baby pig is smaller than its mommy."

Clinician: "Yes, you are right. What's happening in this picture?"

BOX 2-6   *Structured-Elicitation Models*

Forced-choice model: Obligates client to use desired target (high support)
Cloze procedure: Client is provided with information and must complete request for missing language structure (intermediate support)
Preparatory sets: Clinician indirectly demonstrates target so that client must use it in more natural interaction (low support)

Clinicians who use this treatment may adapt various aspects of it for a specific client who exhibits interactions among the sound system and other language components. No specific response accuracy criteria are set for the completion of different treatment goals. Accordingly, testing for generalization is an important adjunct to measure the effectiveness of the treatment because it will furnish data regarding use outside of treatment.

Language-Based Treatment: Conversational Dialogues

Hoffman and Norris have developed remediation procedures for treating phonology in the context of naturalistic language situations (Hoffman, 1992; Hoffman et al., 1990; Norris and Hoffman, 1990). They have stressed that phonology is one aspect of language and that treatment should be conducted within the milieu of language (Hoffman and Norris, 2005; Norris and Hoffman, 2005). Goals of treatment are general in that they specify expansions to the client's phonetic inventory or improving the percentage of consonants that are used correctly. They do not delineate specific sounds or sound classes because treatment change is attributed to the reorganizing properties of the client's neural network. That is, the child receives linguistic input that is dealt with via a theoretical language-processing model proposed by the authors. Hoffman and Norris believe that the language-processing variables are mutually interactive, and this enables the client to change his or her language (of which phonology is an important component).

Some professionals believe that phonological treatment should be conducted within the broader milieu of language. The client receives linguistic input that is used to refine the different components of language.

Research Note

Hoffman and Norris, 2005; Norris and Hoffman, 2005.

Treatment is conducted within the context of clinician and client interactions that are carried out in simulated language situations (Hoffman, 1992). Acting out play schemes, forming narratives about different event and activities, and reading storybooks form the basis for language input to the client. During the presentation of the activities, the clinician guides the client in processing the verbal and nonverbal input through various scaffolding techniques. The scaffolding techniques assist the client in developing more complex language, including improvements in phonology. In addition, the clinician provides appropriate action and language after each of the client's communicative turns to reward the client for engaging in different speech acts and endeavors to elicit more complex language than the client currently uses in conversational speech. An example of the treatment by Hoffman and colleagues (1990) is summarized for the reader in the following sections (Box 2-7).

Language Activities. The clinician presents an activity of interest to the client. For example, the clinician might present a storybook with illustrative pictures and read the story to the client. The clinician uses the pictures and may point to printed words to talk about the story. The characters are introduced, events are described, and the outcome or conclusion of the story is presented to the client through the use of a variety of different language forms. The child is then asked to retell the story to the clinician; Hoffman and associates (1990) suggest that it may be helpful to have the client retell the story to a puppet. During the story retelling, the clinician provides different forms of feedback contingent on each conversational turn, as in the following sections.

Option A. If the child's response is inaccurate, uncertain, or inadequately stated, then the clinician presents a request for clarification. The clinician then provides pertinent information in a restatement, using

---

BOX 2-7 *Summary of Conversational-Dialogues Treatment*

Clinician presents a language activity that is of interest to the client (e.g., a storybook with illustrative pictures). The clinician presents a story and then asks the client to relate the information back to him or her.

Option A: If the client responds inaccurately or inadequately, then the clinician requests clarification and ultimately a restatement of what the client originally provided.

Option B: If the client describes the event appropriately, then the clinician requests a description of yet another event related to the story.

Option C: If the client can describe individual story events in conversational interchanges, then the clinician introduces prompts to help the client incorporate multiple events into his or her responses.

Data from Hoffman PR, Norris JA, Monjure J: Comparison of process targeting and whole language treatments for phonologically delayed preschool children, *Lang Speech Hear Serv Sch* 21:102-109, 1990.

different language forms and generally expanding on the client's original response. The child is then asked to restate what he or she had originally said.

> Clinician: A picture that is part of a story is presented, which depicts a boy helping his father wash the car.

> Client: "That boy driving."

> Clinician: "No, that's not what is going on. The little boy is helping to clean the car so that the family can ride in the car. When the boy is big, he can drive, but he can't drive now. Let's look at the picture again and you tell what is happening."

If the client continues to experience problems with the story line, then the clinician makes additional restatements. However, direct prompting statements such as "No, say, he is washing the car" are not used in the treatment paradigm.

Option B. When the client describes an event appropriately, the clinician follows with a request to describe another event related to the story.

> Clinician: "Yes, the boy is helping his dad clean the car. After they clean the car, they will go for a ride. Where will they go if they take a ride?"

> Client: The client continues to discuss features of the story using various language structures.

Option C. If the client is able to describe individual story events in the conversational interchanges, then the clinician introduces prompts to facilitate the construction of responses that incorporate multiple events. For example, the clinician might identify potential associations among and between different events or characters, discuss cause and effect, speculate what might happen in the story, or talk about the internal feelings of the characters.

> Client: "The daddy is washing the car and the little boy is helping."

> Clinician: "Yes you are right. They are both cleaning the car. When they finish, the family will go for a ride. Tell me some other things about that part of the story."

The rationale underlying this treatment is to provide language input to the child that will foster the development of novel utterances. In each exchange the clinician provides language input that the child must process and then create novel utterances. The authors suggest that this process helps the child develop more complex syntactic, morphological, and phonological units that should culminate in improved language. Stories and other language-rich activities may be recycled to promote more complex language and new activities introduced during treatment. No pass/fail criteria are set for treatment activities; consequently, generalization assessments are an important adjunct to measure the effectiveness of the treatment for the client's sound system disorder.

PHONOLOGICAL PROCESSING APPROACH

In addition to the linguistic approaches discussed previously, some treatment programs target phonological processes (Dean et al., 1995; Hodson, 1989). Some classify the treatment of processes as a phonemic approach, whereas others say this treatment is simply a labeling of a client's errors in different terminology (Bernthal and Bankson, 2004). That is, phonological-process analysis is a descriptive approach that does not identify whether the process is phonetic or phonemic based. Kamhi (2005) suggests that a causal explanation from a phonological-process rationale is not possible, because this type of analysis does not differentiate between errors that may be phonetic or phonemic based. The phonological-process approach targets processes or patterns that the child uses on a consistent basis. Treatment of a process is proposed to affect generalization across a wide class of sounds that are affected by the process. Advocates of phonological-process treatment suggest that processes that most interfere with intelligibility should be early goals of therapy.

Research Note	Some researchers classify phonological-process treatment as a phonemic approach, whereas others argue that such a classification simply labels a client's errors.

Bernthal and Bankson, 2004.

The description of processes may differ because of the specific framework, but process errors may be classified under three primary categories that include syllable structure processes, features contrast processes, and **harmony (assimilation)** processes (Box 2-8; Bernthal and Bankson, 2004). Syllable structure processes are operations that alter the composition of a word or syllable, whereas feature contrasts are substitutions of place or manner features (or of both). Finally, harmony or assimilation is a context-sensitive or coarticulatory change in word or syllable struc-

---

BOX 2-8 *Process Error Categories*

Syllable structure processes: Deletion of final consonants, glottal replacement, weak syllable deletion, cluster reduction
Feature contrast processes: Stopping, affrication, gliding of fricatives, fronting, denasalization, gliding of liquids, vocalization
Harmony or assimilation processes: Prevocalic voicing, final consonant devoicing, velar assimilation, labial assimilation, alveolar assimilation

---

ture. One segment influences the change of another segment to create phonetic symmetry.

Metaphon

The **metaphon approach** targets phonological processes primarily through the use of metalinguistic awareness tasks (Howell and Dean, 1994), with minimal attention to the production of phonemic contrasts. The underlying rationale of the treatment is to facilitate improvements in phonological processing, not articulatory-production skills. That is, the approach targets the development of the client's awareness of sounds and features of the sound system. Dean and colleagues (1995) indicate that treatment targets should be based on linguistic assessment that identifies the client's phonological process errors. Treatment should be carefully monitored so that positive changes in the client's sound system may be documented. The primary goal of treatment is to provide numerous metalinguistic learning opportunities for the client as he or she is introduced to the sound features of the language. The metaphon treatment consists of two phases or segments, and both center on the development of different aspects of linguistic introspection (Box 2-9). The first phase is designed to formulate an awareness of the sound system, introduce the contrastive features of phonemes, and integrate the newly acquired features in the client's phonemic system. The second phase involves transfer and application of the metalinguistic skills acquired in the first phase to communicative situations.

Phase 1: Imagery Concepts

Treatment is initiated by introducing the child to the contrastive properties of phonemes through the use of imagery concepts (Dean et al., 1995; Klein, 1996). The authors label this first step in phase 1 *concept develop-*

BOX 2-9   *Summary of Phases in Metaphon Approach to Treatment*

Phase 1
1. *Concept development:* Clinician uses imagery concepts to introduce the child to the contrastive properties of phonemes.
2. *Sound level:* Clinician asks the client to incorporate the imagery concepts into nonspeech activities.
3. *Phoneme level:* Clinician and client provide contrasting words spontaneously and identify the contrasting features.
4. *Word level:* Clinician presents the client with contrasting word sets and asks the client to identify the target feature of each.

Phase 2
1. Clinician and client take turns choosing a picture card that illustrates one contrast of a minimal pair. Then the clinician reintroduces a phase 1 activity.
2. *Sentence level:* Clinician asks the client to embed contrastive pairs in carrier phrases.

Data from Howell J, Dean EC: *Treating phonological disorders in children: metaphon-theory to practice*, ed 2, London, 1994, Whurr.

ment. For example, a client might substitute stops in place of fricatives, thus exhibiting a stopping process. The imagery concepts of "flowing sounds" versus "dripping sounds" might be used to contrast the production features of fricatives with stops. Similarly, the clinician might instruct the client to "turn on the motor in the throat" for voiced sounds and "turn off the motor in the throat" for voiceless sounds. The contrast might first be introduced by having the client feel the difference by placing the fingers on the area of the thyroid. When the client acquires the imagery distinctions of the target processes, treatment shifts to the second step, which is the referred to as the *sound level.* The client now incorporates the imagery concepts in nonspeech activities. For example, the client might be instructed to blow a toy horn with a long blast to represent the flowing speech sounds and a short blast to contrast with the dripping speech sounds.

The third step in phase 1 is the *phoneme level,* in which the target contrast is presented in the context of words (Howell and Dean, 1994).

Both the clinician and the client produce contrasting words spontaneously and identify the contrasting features. For example, the client is shown a picture card with a depiction of flowing water as a cue to either produce or identify a word containing a fricative. After the response the clinician furnishes appropriate feedback. For example, the correct production of a flowing sound would be followed by feedback such as, "You are correct! That was one of our flowing sounds. Can you think of any other flowing sounds?" Feedback after an incorrect response would consist of feature error identification and an opportunity to furnish a correct response. In a typical treatment sequence, the clinician might say, "Oh, I showed you a picture of a flowing sound, but I heard you make a dripping sound instead. I need you to try to say a flowing sound like /f/ or /s/. Try it now."

The final step in phase 1 is the *word level*—exclusively a perceptual step. The client is given contrasting word sets such as *see-tea*, and he or she is required to identify the target feature of each. The /s/ in the word *see* demonstrates the flowing feature, whereas /t/ in the word *tea* is a sound that has the dripping feature.

Phase 2: Feature Identification and Production

This phase of the treatment is composed of two steps (Howell and Dean, 1994). The first step is a minimal-pairs activity that involves participation from both the clinician and client. They alternately take turns choosing a picture card that illustrates one contrast of the minimal pair. Several pairs are used that share the contrastive feature or features (e.g., *sea-tea, she-key, Tay-Kay*). The card is selected, and the speaker identifies the picture. The listener then specifies which of the contrasts was perceived by pointing to a card that illustrates the feature. In the ongoing example, the listener would point to a card depicting either a flowing sound or a dripping sound.

After the feature identification is completed, a phase 1 activity is reintroduced. For example, correct feature identification by the client might result in the clinician having the client categorize the flowing versus dripping sounds that make up the word pairs and paste them with a picture of flowing or dripping water, whichever is appropriate. An instructional cycle of selecting an item, producing the item, identifying the feature, and reintroducing a phase 1 activity is used.

The final step of phase 2 is a production step that is referred to as the *sentence level*. The contrastive pairs are embedded in carrier phrases that, according to the authors, allow for the transfer of metalinguistic knowledge to more realistic communicative situations. For example, the client

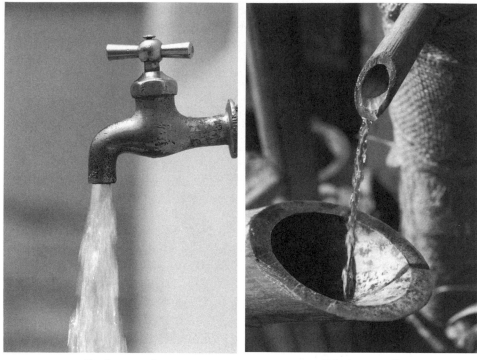

Flowing sound*   Dripping sound*

might use the carrier phrase, "I put the sea/tea on the board." Each activity in phases 1 and 2 is conducted until the clinician judges that the client has acquired the treatment concept; no set accuracy response criteria exist.

Cycles Approach to the Treatment of Phonological Processes

Hodson and associates formulated this treatment, and it has been a very popular for children with severe sound system disorders (Hodson, 1989; Hodson and Paden, 1983). The underlying principle is that cycles are used to develop patterns of intelligible speech. Cycles are time periods that are used to remediate phonological processes or patterns in succession. The authors suggest that the treatment cycles more closely approximate normal phonological acquisition than traditional treatment approaches because this gradual process is somewhat specific among clients. Phonemes within targeted patterns are practiced to achieve acquisition of a particular pattern. Hodson (1989) indicates that the treatment facilitates the formation of new auditory and kinesthetic images that lead to improved client self-monitoring; the purpose is not to establish phonetic motor patterns.

The purpose of cycles treatment is not to establish phonetic motor patterns; rather, the treatment facilitates the formation of new auditory and kinesthetic images that lead to improved client self-monitoring.	*Research* Note

Hodson, 1989.

It is recommended that a phoneme within a pattern be treated individually for at least 60 minutes in a cycle before treating another phoneme of the same pattern. When all phonemes on that pattern are treated, another phonological pattern is introduced. Only one phonological pattern is covered during a single session, thereby enabling the client to focus on the major treatment pattern. At least 2 hours is allotted for a pattern per cycle. The cycle could be anywhere from 5 to 16 weeks in length, depending on the number of patterns or processes that require treatment. The first cycle is to establish productive control of a pattern. After all patterns have been targeted in a cycle, a new cycle is introduced. In succeeding cycles, the child further stabilizes the patterns, and transfer activities to other speaking contexts are used. Usually three to six cycles are used for a client.

The ordering of the patterns depends on the stimulability of the child. That is, the most stimulable targets are chosen first for training so that the client will experience initial success with the treatment. Hodson (1989) indicates that primary patterns should be treated first to assist the client in improving intelligibility. After acquisition of the primary patterns, intervention is directed to secondary targets. A listing of the targets is presented in Box 2-10. Primary targets are early goals of treatment because they have a significant effect on the client's intelligibility. Secondary targets are introduced after the client has suppressed the primary targets; however, the author indicates that treatment of secondary patterns is frequently unnecessary for preschool clients because they exhibit significant phonological generalization. If treatment is necessary for secondary patterns, then Hodson recommends that minimal pairs be used. In addition, some clients may reveal problematic advanced

---

BOX 2-10 *Phonological Patterns That May Be Targeted in the Cycles Treatment Program*

Primary Targets
1. *Syllableness:* Treat syllable structure patterns if client cannot sequence syllables (e.g., baseball, chimney). Treatment is directed to syllable combinations, not exact consonant productions.
2. *Prevocalic singleton consonants:* Treat initial consonant deletions, if early-appearing nasals /m, n/, stops /p, b, t, d/, and the labiopalatal glide /w/ are deleted.
3. *Postvocalic singleton consonants:* Treat postvocalic consonant deletions if voiceless stops /p, t, k/, nasals /m, n/ are deleted, or both occur.
4. *Additional word structures:* Treat CVC (e.g., boat) and VCV (e.g., abby) if problematic for the client. The same consonant configuration may facilitate CVC combinations (e.g., babe).
5. *Fronting and backing:* Treat velar stops /k, g/ if substituted by alveolar stops /t, d/, or treat alveolar stops if substituted by velar stops.
6. */s/ clusters:* Treat /s/ clusters if missing; /s/ clusters should be treated before singleton /s/ in cases of substitution of /t/ for /s/.
7. *Liquids /r, l/:* Liquids should be stimulated during each cycle if not used by the client.

Secondary Targets
1. *Prevocalic voicing:* Voice onset time (VOT) associated with prevocalic voiceless stops is problematic (e.g., *dough* for *toe*).
2. *Vowel neutralization:* Neutral vowel is used place of other vowels (e.g., *putt* for *pat*, *peat*).
3. *Assimilation:* Context-sensitive pattern errors (e.g., *men* for *pen*) must be considered.
4. *Idiosyncratic patterns:* Pattern errors that are reflective of the individual client are targeted.

Data from Hodson BW: Phonological remediation: a cycles approach. In Creaghead NA, Newman PW, Secord WA, editors: *Assessment and remediation of articulatory and phonological disorders*, Columbus, Ohio, 1989, Merrill.

target patterns in the elementary years (e.g., problems producing multisyllabic words). Treatment may be directed to this pattern by noting problematic words and helping the client break down and then combine the segmental components of the problem words. Finally, Hodson recommends that some patterns should not be considered as primary targets in the cycles approach. These include treatment of voiced final obstruent sounds, postvocalic and syllabic /l/, weak syllable deletion, and the linguadental fricatives /θ,ð/.

Cycles Treatment Session (Box 2-11)

Step 1:   The first step in a treatment session is generally a review of the target items used during the previous session (Hodson, 1989). For example, if the client was working on stopping of fricatives pattern, then he or she would review the practice item pictures from the last session and be introduced to new practice items for the current session. Each item would be presented via a picture, and the client would produce the items individually. The clinician would provide feedback regarding response accuracy. If a new pattern was being introduced, then the previous practice items from a different pattern would not be reviewed. Instead they might be saved and used with other practice items during a later cycle.

Step 2:   The second step is an auditory perceptual step that is known as *auditory bombardment*. The practice items for the session are presented to the child through mild amplification. The list of items consists of about 10 to 12 practice words. The child is asked to listen while the clinician presents the items for a short period of time. The clinician also simulates the error pattern and contrasts it with the intended target during the auditory bombardment. After the auditory bombardment has been com-

---

BOX 2-11   *Summary of Steps in Cycles Treatment Approach*

1. Review of target items used in previous session
2. Auditory bombardment
3. Creative activity
4. Experiential play activities
5. Stimulability probes
6. Repeat of auditory bombardment
7. Short daily practice sessions between client and caregiver or school assistant

---

Data from Hodson BW: Phonological remediation: a cycles approach. In Creaghead NA, Newman PW, Secord WA, editors: *Assessment and remediation of articulatory and phonological disorders*, Columbus, Ohio, 1989, Merrill.

pleted, the clinician may request that the client produce one or two potential target items into the microphone of the amplifier. The target items are not from the list of 10 to 12 practice words, but rather items that may be introduced in another session.

Step 3:   The client is engaged in a creative activity during the third step. He or she draws, colors, or pastes three to five pictures on index cards that the clinician has selected. The items are examples of the pattern that is undergoing treatment. The client produces each item before creating the picture so that the clinician may evaluate the item and determine whether the item is suitable for inclusion as a treatment item. The clinician prints the name of each picture on the index cards so that others such as parents may be able to identify the items.

Step 4:   After the picture preparation has been completed, the client is introduced to more concentrated production practice through experiential-play activities. Such activity is designed to motivate the client, provide a more natural context for speech, and permit the clinician to cue the client when targets are produced incorrectly. The monitoring of training trials through charting and graphing performance is not recommended because the author believes that such activity interferes with the naturalness of the experiential-play activities. This step generally requires the largest amount of time within a treatment session.

The clinician needs to select games and activities that are appealing to the client and provide avenues for the production of target items that were introduced previously. For example, a board game that requires the production of target items can be used. The experiential-play activities can be varied, and more than one activity may be used in a session. Models and other cues must be given to facilitate successful elimination of the target pattern. Models and cues help the client to attain correct production, thus eliminating the target pattern. This step is crucial to the success of the treatment regimen. The clinician should also provide opportunities for the client to engage in conversation so that phonological patterns can be monitored for use in spontaneous contexts.

Hodson cautions that practice words should be chosen carefully (particularly during early cycles) to ensure success. Nominals and action words can easily be incorporated in activity themes or games. Initially, the clinician should select monosyllables with facilitative phonetic contexts (Kent, 1982). Words with phonemes at the same place of articulation as the pattern substitution should not be used during early cycles. Words that may trigger assimilation effects should also be avoided.

The clinician should choose practice words carefully, particularly during early cycles. Initially, monosyllables with facilitative phonetic contexts should be used.

Research Note

Hodson, 1989; Kent, 1982.

Step 5: Stimulability probes are conducted after experiential play to identify target patterns for the next session. For example, if /s/ as part of stopping for fricatives is the next target phoneme of pattern suppression, then the clinician would select a group of /s/ words to be used for probing. The child would be asked to watch, listen, and then try to say each individual word. Those /s/ words found to be stimulable would serve as practice items for the next session.

Step 6: The auditory bombardment used in step 2 is repeated with the same word items that were used previously.

Step 7: In this step the child's caregiver or a school assistant conducts short daily practice sessions with the client. The caregiver reads the list of words that were used in auditory bombardment treatment, and the client identifies pictures of the production–practice word items.

The cycles approach is a very popular because it can be used with clients who have severe intelligibility problems. The additional feature is the use of sequencing of treatment cycles so that multiple targets may first be acquired and then stabilized in succeeding cycles, if necessary. Decisions regarding the completion of treatment goals and the introduction of new treatment goals are based on clinical judgment.

PHONETIC TREATMENT APPROACH

The phonetic approach to treatment teaches the motor movements requisite to a particular sound using principles of motor skill learning. In early investigations of sound system intervention, the phonetic aspect of phonology was the driving force in treating clients, and systematic treatment was initially examined with school-aged clients in both empirical and descriptive studies (Diedrich and Bangert, 1980; Elbert et al., 1967). The data show that motor-learning principles were successful in bringing about change in clients with residual sound system errors that were in the moderate to mild range of severity; however, the authors made no claim that the phonetic approach influences phonemic learning. In reality, clear-cut definitive phonetic and phonemic distinctions are difficult to make and remain controversial (Kahmi, 2005; Ruscello, 1993).

Research Note	Studies have shown that motor-learning principles have been successful in facilitating change in clients with residual sound system errors in the moderate to mild range of severity.

Diedrich and Bangert, 1980; Elbert et al., 1967.

The reader should note that motor skill–learning theory forms the foundation for phonetic treatment in this interpretation of traditional sound-by-sound intervention, and phonological theory forms the basis for phonemic contrast. The underlying learning theory for treating phonemic-based disorders is operant learning because it can be used to introduce phonemic contrasts in a systematic and efficient way. Clinicians need to be aware of this theoretical distinction when planning treatment for a specific client. In one case, motor skill–learning theory forms the basis for *what* and *how* to teach phonetic skills, whereas in the other case, operant learning forms the basis for *how* to teach different phonemic contrasts. Readers should refer to Chapter 1 for a discussion of the components of motor skill learning for treatment of phonetic-based sound system disorders.

Phonetic Treatment Activities

If the client is unable to produce the target sound correctly, the starting point in phonetic treatment is at the isolated sound level if phonetically permissible or in the context of a syllable. When correct target sound production has been attained, activities are introduced to integrate the sound in a wide variety of contexts that include nonsense or nonce syllables, words, phrases, and spontaneous conversation. The underlying rationale is to have the client practice systematically under conscious control, with internal feedback and knowledge of results helping him or her to stabilize the target sound. During the initial stages of treatment, the client is asked to *think* about the movements associated with the sound, *plan* the movements, and then *produce* the target. After the target has been acquired, a shift to automated practice without conscious control occurs. The motor skill has been incorporated into the client's repertoire of motor skill routines.

The clinician should also be cognizant of the fact that most descriptions of phonetic treatment introduce levels of practice in a progressive order, which is known as *block sequencing*. That is, the client moves in a progression from isolation through conversation in a stairstep manner. In a motor skill–learning description, levels of treatment also may be randomized and introduced in this manner during each session. All levels of the treatment are randomized and presented during each session. As discussed in Chapter 1, research suggests that random sequencing results in slightly lower accuracy rates during practice sessions; however, greater generalization to nontrained items is seen (Schmidt and Wrisberg, 2000; Skelton, 2004).

Isolation Sound Teaching

Numerous methods exist for teaching the correct production of target sounds (Bernthal and Bankson, 2004; Secord, 1981a; Shriberg, 1975), and the clinician should be systematic when attempting to elicit target sounds. Common methods consist of (1) auditory and visual stimulation (stimulability), (2) **contextual facilitation,** (3) phonetic placement, and (4) shaping.

Stimulability. Stimulability is the ability of the client to produce a target sound in isolation or in a syllable following cues by the clinician, such as "Watch me, listen carefully, and say /s/." Elicitation of the correct target in isolation would then be followed by stimulability trials with the sound in syllables or words. Clients who are able to produce the target sound with auditory and visual cueing are stimulable. Miccio (2005) indicates that stimulability is a positive prognostic indicator, which suggests that the child has sensorimotor control of the target. Stimulable sounds are likely to improve without intervention; however, stimulable sounds are frequently targets for treatment in the phonetic approach.

Miccio (2005) argues that stimulability also be used as a therapeutic agent to expand the client's phonetic inventory. Children with limited phonetic inventories could benefit from such a program because it aids expansion and stimulable sounds are likely to demonstrate generalization. Rather than simply assess stimulability before initiating treatment, the clinician implements a stimulability program as part of the client's treatment. Miccio developed the following program to promote stimulability (Box 2-12):

Step 1: The clinician assesses stimulability at the isolation and syllable levels (CV) to identify stimulable and nonstimulable sounds. Nonstimulable sounds are selected for intervention.

BOX 2-12 *Summary of Steps in Stimulability Promotion*

1. Stimulability assessment at isolation and syllable levels
2. Teaching of nonstimulable sounds in isolation or syllables, matching of each sound with object, and drawing of objects
3. Probing for nonstimulable sounds at beginning of each session
4. Presentation of all pictures individually
5. Interactive-play activities

Data from Miccio AW: A treatment program for enhancing stimulability. In Kamhi AG, Pollock KE, editors: *Phonological disorders in children*, Baltimore, 2005, Paul H Brookes.

Step 2:   Nonstimulable sounds are taught in isolation or syllables. For instance, "Billy, watch me and say f:::::::" or "Billy, watch me and say puh." This author recommends that the stimuli be produced at a normal loudness level without extensive facial exaggeration. Each sound is matched with a character that represents an animal or object, and the characters are drawn or pictures are placed on index cards. A specific body motion or hand gesture is also paired with the sound. For example, /f/ is *fussy fish,* and the associated body motion is to *fussily push hand away from body.*

Step 3:   At the initiation of each session, a probe is conducted for the nonstimulable sounds. Each target is sampled in isolation and the syllable contexts of CV, VCV, and VC with the vowel /i/. During the next session the vowel /a/ is used, and at the next session /u/ is used. The vowels are recycled in order as treatment continues. A brief word probe is also administered at the end of the session, which targets the sounds in CVC contexts (e.g., fife, sauce).

Step 4:   After administration of the probe, all pictures including stimulable and nonstimulable sounds are presented individually, with the sound and associated hand and body motion by the clinician. The clinician must ensure that the client is attending to the task when each sound is presented.

Step 5:   Treatment is conducted via interactive-play activities that offer the client numerous opportunities to imitate the target sounds. Stimulable and nonstimulable sounds are included so that the client will experience success during the course of a treatment session. For instance, the clinician and client may play a matching game of concentration with the character cards. A match would involve production of the target with the paired hand and body motion. The clinician furnishes the appropriate verbal knowledge of results to the client for a correct response. The clinician also acknowledges incorrect responses because the associated hand motion can be used to decipher them. The clinician can then recue the client to attempt production of the nonstimulable target sound. As an example, the client may not produce /f/ correctly, but the clinician is aware of the target by the associated hand movement or body movement. The clinician could then follow with "Maybe I have fussy fish. Let me look. I found it. Fussy fish makes the sound /f::::::/, doesn't it? Yes it does, it says /f::::::/." When the child becomes at ease with the stimulability treatment and imitates the clinician, additional cues can be introduced. For instance, the client can be cued to watch the clinician, listen, and say the target sound, or the attention cues can be presented in conjunction with phonetic placement cues.

Contextual Facilitation. Some clients produce target sounds correctly on an inconsistent basis; on assessment, the differences in production accuracy are attributed to contextual influences (Kent, 1982). McDonald (1964) maintains that most clients demonstrate such inconsistencies, and the variations can be identified through contextual testing. This notion of contextual facilitation has resulted in the development of the Deep Test of Articulation and a phonetic treatment program known as the *Sensory-Motor Approach*, which was introduced by McDonald (McDonald, 1964; Shine, 1989). That is, phonetic environments exist in which the client's target productions are perceived as being produced correctly. McDonald (1964) and Secord (1981b) developed specific protocols to identify potential contexts. Treatment stimuli that are constructed on the basis of different phonetic contexts are also available and may be used by the reader (Griffiths and Miner, 1979; Secord and Shine, 1997).

Some clients demonstrate inconsistencies in the production of correct target sounds, and the variations can be identified through contextual testing.

Research Note

McDonald, 1964.

Kent (1982) discussed contextual facilitation and conducted a review of the literature. His findings are summarized as follows for consideration in treatment (Box 2-13):

- Target sounds should be embedded in stressed syllables. Stressed syllables ensure that the articulations are distinct and clearly articulated. Kent (1982) also indicates that stressed syllables provide a well-defined acoustic model that allows the clinician to judge the accuracy of practice targets.
- Word position may have a facilitating effect on the client's productions. Initial syllable /Cr/ clusters such as /tr/, /dr/, and /gr/ are frequently facilitative for /r/ (McCauley and Skenes, 1987). Similarly, the medial or final position of words is often facilitative for correct /s/ productions. Kent also points out that some phonemes such as /r/ and /l/ show different allophonic variation as a function of position. For instance, prevocalic /r/ is produced with more lip rounding, a more frontal tongue location, and a lesser amount of dorsal tongue grooving than its postvocalic variant.
- The influence of bordering sounds in some cases can be facilitative. Contextual arrangements such as /sp/, /st/, and /sn/ in prevocalic clusters have been identified as facilitative for /s/.
- Kent advises clinicians to consider syllable stress, word position, and adjacent sounds in trying to find contexts that support correct target sound production. In some cases, contexts will be identified and serve as a basis for the initial stages of treatment. The clinician would work from facilitating contexts to nonfacilitating contexts. One final caution is that error type has not really been considered in this research, but

---

BOX 2-13 *Summary of Contextual Facilitation Findings*

Target sounds should be embedded in stressed syllables.

Word position may have a facilitating effect on the client's production.

Influence of abutting sounds can sometimes be facilitative.

Clinicians should consider syllable stress, word position, and adjacent sounds in trying to find contexts that support correct target sound production.

Variation of a bite block may be used to isolate the jaw from the lips and tongue when trying to identify facilitative contexts.

Data from Kent RD: Contextual facilitation of correct sound production, *Lang Speech Hear Serv Sch* 13:66-76, 1982.

the reader is advised to consider error type. For example, a client with an /s/ error of lateralization may differ from a client with an /s/ error of dentalization in his or her response to facilitating agents.

- A variation of a bite block may be used to isolate the jaw from the lips and tongue when trying to identify facilitative contexts. A tongue blade may be inserted between the upper and lower canines. Netsell (1985) suggests that the width of the blade be trimmed to approximately 5 to 8 mm for children. The client is instructed to bite down gently on the blade. With stabilization of the jaw, alveolar and velar points of articulation may be examined in the context of different consonant and vowel environments.

Stressed syllables provide well-defined acoustic models that allow the clinician to judge the accuracy of practice targets.

Research Note

Kent, 1982.

Phonetic Placement. One of the most frequently used techniques for eliciting sounds is **phonetic placement.** Secord (1989) indicates that clinicians use verbal instructions, illustrations, and different types of feedback to acquire correct target sound production. For instance, the clinician instructs the client, "I want you to place your tongue behind your front teeth and smile while you make an /s/ sound." The verbal instructions might also be used in conjunction with a diagram that depicts the placement of /s/. The client receives verbal placement instructions that are paired with a diagram of the target sound. Different sensory feedback is also used, such as observing one's productions via a mirror, sensing voicing and voicelessness with the fingers placed on the thyroid cartilage, and placing the articulators in position with the fingers or a tongue blade. If phonetic placement is to be used, then the clinician should know the production features of the phonemes to be taught. Incorrect placement information or sensory feedback can hamper a client's potential for correct target sound production. Different phonetic placement techniques can be found in the literature (Bernthal and Bankson, 2004; Secord, 1981a).

Verbal instructions, illustrations, and different types of feedback are all used in phonetic placement.

Research Note

Secord, 1989.

Shaping. This sound-teaching technique consists of isolating the components of a phoneme and teaching the components individually or shaping from a sound that the client has in his or her inventory (Secord, 1989). The components of a phoneme are then incorporated to obtain the desired target sound. For example, the clinician might teach the client elements of a sound and then combine them to produce the target. A client with dentalization of /s/ would be taught, "Close your teeth and make sure that your tongue is behind the teeth. Let me see you do it." The client practices the movement, and then the clinician adds another element. "Close your teeth and make sure that your tongue is behind the teeth. Now I want you to smile. Let me see you do it." When the second element is mastered, a third is added. "Close your teeth and make sure that your tongue is behind the teeth. Now I want you to smile and make the /s::::::/ like this. Let me see you do it." This type of isolation treatment is designed to allow a gradual approximation to achieving correct target sound production.

Shaping from a sound in the client's inventory to a target sound can be done in a variety of ways. For instance, the clinician can shape /s/ from the linguadental /θ/ by instructing the client to produce /θ/ and prolong the production. While gradually prolonging /θ/, the client is instructed to place the tongue behind the teeth and keep it there to change the production from /θ/ to /s/. Another example is establishing the voiced and voiceless distinction for **cognates.** The client is told, "I want you to make the /z/ sound in a different way. Make it, but make it with a whisper. Listen carefully, you are making /s/ when you whisper."

In summary, some clients cannot produce the target sound, and they are taught to produce it in isolation or in a syllable. The most frequently used elicitation techniques are sound stimulation, contextual facilitation, phonetic placement, and shaping. They can be used individually or in combination, but the clinician should also include a mental focus to the treatment. For instance, the client can be instructed to rehearse mentally before producing the target sound (cues such as "We make the /f/ sound by touching our bottom lip with our top teeth and then blowing air. Think about the sound and then make it like this /f::::::/"). Limited research exists regarding the effectiveness of isolation sound treatment, but a study by Wingo and Hoshiko (1972) indicates that the most effective elicitation techniques in descending order are (1) sound stimulation, (2) phonetic placement instructions, (3) the combination of sound stimulation and phonetic placement instructions, and (4) positioning of the articulators. Contextual facilitation and shaping were not studied. As previously emphasized, if a client needs isolation treatment for sounds that are absent from the phonetic inventory, then the clinician must be aware of the production characteristics of the phoneme or phonemes.

The most effective elicitation techniques in descending order are sound stimulation, phonetic placement instructions, and positioning of articulators. Contextual facilitation and shaping were not studied.

Research Note

Wingo and Hoshiko, 1972.

Syllables and Words

Syllables and words represent the initial use of the target in context, but researchers presume that these levels of practice continue to require conscious control on the part of the learner (Ruscello, 1993). That is, the learner must be encouraged to continue to "think about, plan, and evaluate" the production movements of the target sound when using it in a syllable or word. The client is asked to focus on the required movements of the target sound, plan those movements, and then evaluate the results. The internally focused activities do not have to be carried out for each response, rather they are interspersed throughout practice at syllable and word levels. Theses are metaphonological skills that may exceed the developmental level of preschool clients; consequently, the clinician should use them with school-aged clients (Justice and Schuele, 2004). The examples in Box 2-14 illustrate the use of focus on target sound production. The reader should note that syllable practice is not requisite to word practice; the clinician may introduce words and not use syllable practice activities with a particular client.

Generally the training trials at this level are designed initially to develop imitative control of the target sound. The clinician models syllables and words, and the client is expected to imitate the models. After imitative control has been achieved, training shifts to more spontaneous elicitation cues. For example, the first practice condition might be direct imitation or modeling, followed by direct modeling paired with the picture of the practice item, followed by presentation of the picture alone. In this way the clinician builds a response that is more resistant to reversion of the former incorrect response, and it can be elicited in conditions that approximate spontaneous production of the target. Generally the practice activities are carried out in a drill or drill/play manner

---

BOX 2-14   *Sample Training Trial Illustrating a Mental Practice Feature*

Sample Training Trial 1
Clinician: "I want you to think really hard about your new sound before you say the word. Remember to put your tongue behind your front teeth for /s/, and make sure that your tongue does not stick out. Think about it and then say the word *soup*."
Client: "Soup."
Clinician: "Good job"

Sample Training Trial 2
Clinician: "I want you to think really hard about your new sound before you say the word. Remember to put your tongue behind your front teeth for /s/, and make sure that your tongue does not stick out. Think about it and then say the word *soup*."
Client: "Soup."
Clinician: "Did you make the new /s/ sound in the word?
Client: "Yes, I did."
Clinician: "You did, great job!"

---

because the treatment is formulated to facilitate active participation and repetitive practice.

The target sound may be juxtaposed in different syllable and word shapes (e.g., CV, VC, CVC, VCV, CCV, CVCCVC), which depend on the client's needs. If interference from the error is seen, then nonce syllables can be used to ease the transition from isolation to context. A nonce syllable is a practice unit with an attached meaning that is novel to the child; consequently a nonce syllable is not as likely to trigger an error response (see Chapter 1 for examples).

Phrases and Sentences

Practice at phrase and sentence levels signals the transition from conscious internal or mental focus to activities intended to automate the target sound in context (Ruscello, 1993). Clinicians may choose to bypass phrases and move directly to sentences, which is a clinical judgment. Presumably, the client no longer needs to rely extensively on internal feedback and knowledge of results information provided by the clinician. Words with the target sound are integrated into phrase- and sentence-level materials. It may be necessary to begin at the imitative level, but this should be quickly phased out in favor of more spontaneous methods such as having the client respond to pictures, printed material, picture stories, and sequenced activities. The sentence material can be graded in terms of sentence length, number of target words, and complexity of target words. For instance, initial responses may require a short sentence containing a single target word embedded in a simple syllable shape. This is followed by longer sentences, multisyllabic target words, the target in a cluster, and more than one target word in a sentence. Although the activities at this level are designed to automate the target sound, the clinician should periodically have the client evaluate some of his or her phrase or sentence responses to continue self-monitoring activities (Koegel et al., 1986).

In addition to regular practice activities with phrases and sentences, other practice activities can be used to automate target production. Speed drills, practice under auditory masking, and rehearsal matrices are additional automating activities that can be interspersed during treatment (Ruscello, 1993). **Speed drills** consist of material that is produced by the client in practice sets across a number of training trials with a gradual reduction in the time necessary to practice the material. For instance, the clinician may construct a list of 15 sentences, and the client is instructed to read the sentences and use the target sound correctly. The time needed to read the sentences and the accuracy rate for the practice set is recorded. The client is then instructed to read the sentence list in less time, while maintaining the accuracy rate. The time and accuracy rate are measured, and the results are discussed with the client. Additional sets can be conducted with the goal of reducing time and sustaining the accuracy rate. The speed drills may also be carried out with words or phrases, if the clinician chooses to do so.

During treatment, additional automating activities such as speed drills, practice under auditory masking, and rehearsal matrices can be interspersed to help automate target production.

Research Note

Ruscello, 1993.

Originally, Manning and colleagues (1976) developed auditory masking as a method to assess the automatic use of a target sound. The following description is a treatment variation:

• The client reads a list of words, phrases, or sentences containing the target sound, and an accuracy rate is established.

- The client is then told that he or she will read the material again, but will wear a headset and noise will be played while reading. Masking noise from an audiometer can be recorded and the recording played through a headset while the client is engaged in the production task.
- Comparison of accuracy rates between the masking and nonmasking conditions is then performed and discussed with the client.
- The final activity, rehearsal matrices, is one that was reported by Hoffman and colleagues (1989). Rehearsal matrices are different consonant-vowel nonsense syllable combinations that provide various contextual practice contexts. Clients practice the matrices without morphosyntactic or semantic constraints. A flip chart can be prepared, which allows the clinician to present different contextual combinations for practice. A summary of automation activities is presented in Table 2-2.

Conversation

The final practice condition is conversation. The clinician creates opportunities for the client to use the target sound in spontaneous speech. Generally this is the terminal goal of therapy—correct and automatic use of the target sound in conversation. As with phrase and sentence practice, conversational tasks are presented along a continuum of more structure or clinician control to less structure or minimal control. At

Table 2-2
Activities Used in Target Sound Automation

ACTIVITY	DESCRIPTION
Speed drill	Timed drills are used to reduce practice time but maintain accuracy
Auditory masking	Client practices under conditions of nonmasking and masking; accuracy rates are compared among tasks
Rehearsal matrices	Different phonetic contexts are used for practice (see example)
	VC VCV CV VCCV is isi si itsi es ese se etse

first, structured tasks are used to obtain target responses in conversation. For instance, the clinician may present a sequenced picture story that contains target items. The child is given a picture and discusses that portion of the story using the target word or words. The client is able to anticipate production of the target in the structured tasks; this functions as a transition step from sentences to conversation. As the client's phonetic target skills improve, less structured conversational tasks are presented. For example, the clinician introduces topic cards that are used to stimulate conversation. The client selects a topic card and discusses the topic. Target words cannot be anticipated because the task is less structured and the client is generating the conversation. Numerous activities can be used to generate narratives or conversational interchanges between the client and clinician (Secord, 1989). The spontaneity of the conversational tasks requires automatic production of target sounds in connected speech.

TO SUM UP

In this chapter the phonetic approach is discussed under the guise of motor skill learning, although other theoretical descriptions of phonetic approaches exist (Secord, 1989; Shine, 1989). It is posited that the learner passes through stages of phonetic skill development. Development of phonetic responses occurs as a function of practice, and practice activities differ in reference to the stages of response development. Acquisition activities allow the client to focus mentally on the task and carry out guided practice that is subject to internal feedback and external knowledge of results. After acquisition, activities are presented to automate the phonetic target sound in more spontaneous situations. Less reliance on feedback and knowledge of results is seen, and more emphasis is placed on incorporating the target in a variety of communication situations. Box 2-15 summarizes the various phonetic treatment activities.

BOX 2-15 *Phonetic Treatment Activities*

Isolation sound teaching
    Stimulability
    Contextual facilitation
    Phonetic placement
    Shaping
Syllables and words
Phrases and sentences
Conversation

HYBRID APPROACHES

Representation-Based Approach

Rvachew (2005) formulated this treatment, which encompasses auditory perception, phonetic practice, and phonemic contrast in the treatment of clients with sound system disorders. Because these features reflect a combination of different program elements, the author of this text classifies the treatment advocated by Rvachew as a *hybrid approach* (Box 2-16). The first phase of the treatment is one of phonemic perception and stimulability training. The perceptual-phonetic production phase is followed by a phonemic phase of minimal-pairs contrast using words and short phrases. Finally, the third phase is one that involves phonetic practice of the target or targets in sentences, spontaneous conversation, and narratives.

Phase 1: Phoneme Perception and Phonetic Training

The author indicates that children with speech sound disorders frequently have problems of perception of fine-grained phonemic contrasts as found with liquid and fricative speech sounds (Rvachew, 2005). Research by Rvachew and her associates (Rvachew, 1994; Rvachew and Jamieson, 1989; Rvachew et al., 1999) suggest that a client's errors of perception and production are symptomatic of a disparity between the client's phonological knowledge and the adult organization of underly-

---

BOX 2-16 *Summary of Phases in the Representation-Based Treatment Approach*

Phase 1: Phoneme Perception and Phonetic Training
Perception training using Speech Assessment and Interactive Learning System (SAILS)
Introduction of stimulability teaching

Phase 2: Phonemic Treatment with Minimal Pairs
Introduction of phonemic contrasts

Phase 3: Phonetic Transfer
Practice phase in which client incorporates target in sentences, conversation, and narration

---

Data from Rvachew S: The importance of phonetic factors in phonological intervention. In Kamhi AG, Pollock KE, editors: *Phonological disorders in children*, Baltimore, 2005, Paul H Brookes.

ing phonological contrasts. To assist in the development of phoneme contrasts that are targeted for treatment, perception training is carried out using a computer program, known as *Speech Assessment and Interactive Learning System* (SAILS; Avaaz Innovations, 1994). The program consists of different sections targeting speech sounds that young clients frequently misarticulate. The target sound is embedded in the pre- or postvocalic position of a word, and the number of target examples range from 10 to 30 tokens. The stimuli were audio recorded from adults and children to provide the listener with different examples of the word. The stimuli include variations along a continuum of correct to incorrect productions and are designed to aid the client in discriminating allophonic variants in the appropriate phonemic category from those productions that are not in the phonemic category. The author does not set a specific response accuracy criterion but recommends that the child be able to identify correct and incorrect tokens at a high accuracy level before terminating perceptual treatment.

Research suggests that a client's errors of perception and production are symptomatic of a disparity between the client's phonological knowledge and the adult organization of underlying phonological contrasts.

Research Note

Rvachew, 1994; Rvachew and Jamieson, 1989; Rvachew et al., 1999.

The second part of this phase is the introduction of stimulability teaching with the intended target or targets (Miccio, 2005). Rvachew (2005) indicates that general sound elicitation techniques such as sound stimulation, phonetic placement, and shaping should be used if necessary to develop correct production of the target (Secord, 1981a). The author recommends that the initial phase of treatment be terminated when the client achieves 80% to 90% correct imitative control of the target sound or sounds at the syllable or word level in a variety of phonetic contexts. This is to ensure that a client has acquired the appropriate phonetic skills required for the next phase of treatment.

Phase 2: Phonemic Treatment with Minimal Pairs

Phonemic contrasts are introduced during this phase using procedures similar to those described in the previous discussion of minimal pairs. The author indicates that this part of the treatment should not require much time if the client has successfully completed the initial phase and achieved high accuracy levels in perceptual identification and imitative practice. Rvachew indicates that most children pass through this stage very quickly, reaching response accuracy levels of 80% and above for daily treatment sessions; however, she identifies a few exceptions (i.e., clients who tend to overgeneralize and use the target sound in place of the nonerror pair *run-one → run-run*, or clients who develop the contrast but the new sound production is perceived as distorted). In both cases the author combines both the first and second treatment phases for some of the subsequent treatment sessions. Clients are reintroduced to the perceptual training and stimulability teaching in combination with the minimal-pair contrasts.

Phase 3: Phonetic Transfer

The final phase is a practice phase that incorporates the target or targets in sentences, conversation, and different forms of narration. The client is undergoing a restructuring of the underlying representations of those lexical items that contain the target or target's phoneme. The restructuring is achieved by varied practice in the spontaneous contexts discussed. Rvachew (2005) advocates the use of varied activities so that the child has numerous opportunities to use new sounds. Books, art activities, the creation of written or picture narratives, and the use of computer software are examples of contexts for treatment. The client should be exposed to a variety of activities that require the use of new targets across different lexical items. This phase can also be a time in which the clinician attends to any morphosyntax errors that the client displays. In addition, phonological awareness activities may also be introduced in the therapy milieu.

Research Note	Varied activities, such as those involving books, art, creative written or picture narratives, and the use of computer software, help to ensure numerous opportunities for the client to use new sounds.

Rvachew, 2005.

Rvachew (2005) indicates that the monitoring of training trials and generalization testing are also important components of the treatment. The clinician needs these data to make decisions concerning the completion of a phase and introduction of a new phase. The client's performance data are also used to determine when therapy should be terminated and periodic monitoring instituted. A study conducted by McKercher and colleagues (1995) is cited by Rvachew to provide guidelines for dismissal from treatment. Their data suggest that clients who achieve a word accuracy level of 75% or better on a generalization measure may be dismissed from treatment and need only to be monitored periodically.

Collaborative Treatment Approach

Bowen and Cupples (1999, 2004) present another treatment for sound system disorders that the author of this text classifies as a hybrid approach. This broad-based approach consists of components similar to other treatments, but it also includes caregiver roles, phonological awareness, and the block scheduling of treatment sessions. The elements of their treatment include (1) family education, (2) phonological awareness tasks, (3) phonetic production practice, (4) minimal-pairs contrast and auditory bombardment, and (5) home practice (Box 2-17). This comprehensive approach to treatment is based on the premise that clients with phonological disorders need to be directed along the path of normal development, with caregivers directly involved in the process. Moreover, normal phonological acquisition is acquired gradually and is individual to each child. The authors indicate that the treatment differs from other treatments in terms of three key factors. First, it includes an educational module for caregivers, which is presented in an innovative manner. Second, it uses block scheduling so that clients alternate between treatment and treatment breaks. Third, it uses five intervention components (or elements) that compose a unique treatment approach.

Element 1: Family Education and Involvement

Bowen and Cupples (1999) indicate that well-informed caregivers play an important role in the treatment of their children. Initially, caregivers need information concerning their child's sound system disorder; that information consists of both verbal discussion and written information: What is the problem? How does it affect the child's ability to be understood by others? What will be done in treatment? Will I be involved in my child's therapy? What do I need to do to help my child? Bowen (1998) prepared an informational booklet for parents. The information in the pamphlet includes (1) a definition of sound system disorders within a developmental perspective of sound acquisition, (2) a discussion of the assessment and treatment process, (3) a list of questions parents frequently ask, and (4) intervention techniques such as modeling and promoting self-monitoring (discussed along with the role that these facilitation techniques play in parental involvement).

The authors stress that the initial contact with the client's caregiver is very important in forming a successful bond between the caregiver and clinician. Parents are generally in an information-seeking role and need

> **BOX 2-17** *Summary of Elements in Collaborative Treatment Approach*
>
> 1. Family education and involvement
> 2. Phonological awareness tasks, such as the following:
>   Metaphonetic activities
>   Phoneme-grapheme relationships
>   Onset phoneme segmentation matching
>   Rhyme and alliteration awareness
>   Improving the awareness of words in context
>   Phonemic analysis and synthesis
> 3. Phonetic-production skills
> 4. Multiple-exemplar training, such as the following:
>   Client must point to picture clinician produces
>   Client must produce target word, and clinician gives client
>   picture of target item
>   Clinician and client exchange roles
> 5. Home treatment
>   Parent education
>   Metalinguistic training
>   Phonetic-production training
>   Multiple-exemplar training
>   Homework

Data from Bowen C, Cupples L: Parents and children together (PACT): a collaborative approach to phonological therapy, *Int J Lang and Commun Disord* 34:35-55, 1999; Bowen C, Cupples L: The role of families in optimizing phonological therapy outcomes, *Child Lang Teach Ther* 20:245-260, 2004.

to understand the nature of their child's sound system problem. During the early stages of treatment, they will observe portions of the treatment session to understand what is being done with the child. This also provides an informal introduction to what they may do with their child in home practice sessions. After each session, some of the intervention activities are sent home with the client so that the parents can conduct home practice.

Element 2: Phonological-Awareness Tasks

The authors believe that the client should develop self-monitoring skills and that the development of these skills is facilitated through the use of various phonological-awareness tasks. The use of phonological-awareness tasks furnishes opportunities for the client, clinician, and caregivers to engage in language introspection. The client can experiment with his or her language in ways that help in learning about language with an emphasis of the phonological component. The different activities range from sound recognition and discrimination of target sounds to incorporation of targets in various morphophonemic alterations. Justice and Schuele (2004) recommend that the tasks be integrated into therapy, rather than being separate from treatment activities. The following are examples of the activities:

- *Metaphonetic activities:* These activities are designed to introduce the client to treatment targets. For example, the clinician might describe the phonetic production characteristics of the sound and make the sound while instructing the client to watch and listen. Another task might have the client listen to words produced by the clinician, and then the client identifies those words that contain the target sound. Finally, the client is given correct and incorrect tokens produced by the clinician, and he or she must discriminate correct versus incorrect productions.

- *Phoneme-grapheme relationships:* Clients are taught the similarities and differences between phonemes and their graphic counterparts. For example, the phoneme /p/ corresponds to the grapheme *p*, and /s/ corresponds to the grapheme *s*. However, the grapheme *s* also is produced as /z/ in phonologically conditioned morphemes such as *pigs*. The clinician can use an alphabet chart to illustrate the target sound and its incorporation in practice words. Other activities may include labeling pictures of practice materials and having the client underline the target sound, or assisting children in creating stories that contain words with the target sound.

- *Onset phoneme segmentation matching:* Clients are engaged in activities that require the identification and selection of a phoneme that is in the initial position of words. For example, they may be introduced to the target phoneme /r/ and need to select those words that contain /r/ in the initial word position. Choices include both target words and foils. After identification, the client produces the word containing the target sound.

- *Rhyme and alliteration awareness:* The clinician exposes the child to rhyme awareness through the use of different word rhymes and different alliteration patterns. Alliteration is the awareness of phoneme commonalities across two words. For instance, a word pair such as *pat-peach* shares a common sound in the initial word position. Books and various clinician-generated materials serve as sources for presenting different rhyming and alliteration activities.

- *Improving the awareness of words in context:* Phrase- and sentence-level practice materials may also be used for awareness purposes. Justice and Schuele (2004) propose that clients point to individual written words in practice materials to build an awareness of spoken words and their written form and that boundaries exist between written and spoken words.
- *Phonemic analysis and synthesis:* The development of analysis and synthesis skills enables the child to segment (analysis) words into their phonemic components and blend or combine a given phoneme sequence (synthesis) into syllables and words. During therapy production activities, clinicians can engage in analysis and synthesis tasks with clients. For instance, the clinician might segment a practice word and discuss the position of the target within the word, or he or she may blend the phonemic segments and emphasize the target sound.

Clinicians should note that phonological awareness develops on a continuum that begins with the child's awareness of words, then syllables, and finally an awareness of phonemes. Justice and Schuele (2004) indicate that word and syllable awareness are acquired initially and represent shallow levels of awareness; however, phoneme awareness represents a deep or high level of phonological awareness. Word awareness begins as the young child becomes sensitive to rhyme and alliteration. Words are distinct units that are subject to introspective phonological analysis. Syllable awareness includes awareness that multisyllable words contain syllable combinations and that the syllable is composed of phonemic units. In English, **syllable structure** can be identified in terms of onset-rime patterns. Onset is the consonant or cluster combination that occurs before the vowel in the word, whereas rime is the vowel nucleus and those consonants after the vowel. For example, the onset of the word *spot* is *sp*, and the rime is *ot*. Phonemic awareness is a later-developing skill that appears during early school age and coincides with the development of reading skills. Some developmental guidelines are included for treatment and summarized in Table 2-3.

Research Note	Phonological awareness is acquired on a continuum. Word and syllable awareness are acquired initially and represent shallow levels of awareness; phoneme awareness represents a deep level of phonological awareness. As a child becomes sensitive to rhyme and alliteration, word awareness takes shape.

Justice and Schuele, 2004.

Table 2-3
Summary of Phonological Awareness Skills

PHONOLOGICAL AWARENESS SKILL	ESTIMATED AGE OF DEVELOPMENT
Awareness of words	Emerges between 2 and 3 years of age
Awareness of rhyme	Begins to emerge at 2 and continues refinement up to age 5
Awareness of alliteration	Emerges at 3 years of age and continues refinement up to age 5
Awareness of syllables	Acquired between 4 and 5 years of age
Awareness of phonemes	Emerges between 6 and 7 years of age
Phonemic analysis and synthesis	Begins to emerge at 6 and continues refinement up to age 10

Data from Justice LM, Schuele CM: Phonological awareness: description, assessment, and intervention. In Bernthal JE, Bankson NW, editors: *Articulation and phonological disorders*, ed 5, Boston, 2004, Allyn & Bacon.

Element 3: Phonetic-Production Skills

Bowen and Cupples (1999, 2004) acknowledge that some clients need phonetic-production training as part of their treatment. From their perspective, clients with severe sound system disorders may need phonetic training early in treatment to assist in expanding their limited inventories. They also recommend phonetic training for clients with mild impairments because it may be sufficient to trigger the formation of expected phonological patterns. Phonetic placement techniques and sound stimulation are typically used to establish production at the isolation or syllable level, depending on the target sound or sounds. Additional phonetic practice with word units is used but limited (the authors believe that expanded phonetic practice may be detrimental to phonemic development). Most of their clients receive direct treatment to establish phonetic production of target sounds, and approximately 50%

engage in limited phonetic production at word level or other levels of practice in conjunction with phonological awareness tasks. The remaining 50% participate in phonetic drill activities before participating in phonemic treatment activities.

Element 4: Multiple-Exemplar Training

This step in the intervention regimen combines minimal-pairs contrast and auditory perceptual stimulation as the phonemic portion of the treatment. The authors suggest that the auditory perceptual stimulation is similar to the auditory bombardment advocated by Hodson and Paden (1983), but no amplification is used. Minimal-pairs contrasts are introduced in the context of drill/play activities and initially modeled for the client until he or she can respond spontaneously to the picture stimuli. Pictures with the printed word are typically used as stimulus items, and approximately three to nine training pairs are used. The drill activities vary, and some examples include the following:

- The client is instructed to point to the picture produced by the clinician. The minimal pairs are presented individually in random order. For instance, "Point to big, point to cub, point to cup, point to pig."
- The clinician instructs the client to produce a target word, and the clinician responds by giving the client the picture of the target item. If the child produces an incorrect target, then he or she is given that item to create a communication mismatch, or what Weiner (1981) refers to as *homonymy confrontation.*
- The clinician and client exchange roles in this therapy activity. The clinician produces a target item while pointing to the picture, and the client must judge the correctness of the item. The clinician may correctly produce the target or the other minimal pair so that the client must monitor carefully the clinician's productions.

The auditory stimulation activities are used to provide experience with a particular target in an explicit word position, specific phonetic feature, or minimal-contrast word pairs. For example, a list of 10 to 15 words that feature /f/ in the initial word position or minimal pairs that contrast the omission of final consonants can be assembled. The list may be composed of familiar or unfamiliar words and is presented from one to three times per session. The client is instructed to listen carefully while the clinician produces the words.

The components of the treatment are not used for a specific amount of time and can vary in terms of order, but a typical intervention session may consist of the following activities:

1. Auditory stimulation of the minimal-pair contrasts is performed.
2. Minimal-pair contrast activities are introduced.
   a. Client produces different minimal-treatment pairs.
   b. Client judges accuracy of clinician's productions in homonymy confrontation task.
3. Phonetic treatment is provided for a target that will be introduced at a later treatment session.
4. A phonological awareness activity is introduced. The client and clinician view minimal-pair pictures that will be the focus of the next therapy session. The clinician produces each item for the child and prints the word on each picture.
5. Auditory stimulation is carried out again.
6. The parent is given a short summary of the session.
7. Home treatment activities are discussed with the parent who is conducting them.

Element 5: Home Treatment

Home treatment provided by caregivers is the final and an equally important element of the overall home program. Although most treatments discuss the use of caregivers, Bowen and Cupples (1999, 2004) have included caregiver participation as a major element in the treatment process. They believe that active participation in the treatment process has many advantages such as facilitating generalization, demonstrating positive outcomes of treatment, and promoting client and parent interactions in the absence of the clinician. Moreover, the National Outcome Measurement System (NOMS) has identified the advantage of home treatment conducted by caregivers with their children.

The authors recommend that home practice be carried out approximately 5 to 6 days per week. Parent-child practice sessions should be carried out one to three times per day for about 5 to 7 minutes. Home practice activities consist of perceptual training, production practice, and phonological awareness tasks with an emphasis on perceptual training and awareness tasks. Although caregivers may want to emphasize production tasks, the authors believe that auditory perceptual training and awareness tasks should be given priority. The clinician prepares a homework book for the client that contains an outline of home activities for each week. The clinician and caregiver review these before enactment at home so that the caregiver understands the nature of the tasks and their requirements. This is also done to train the caregiver in the technical aspects of the home treatment such as presentation of stimuli, evaluation of stimuli, provision of appropriate feedback, and collection of data. The components of the parent program are as follows:

- *Parent education:* Parents are introduced to teaching techniques such as modeling, recasting, and feedback strategies that they will use with their child.
- *Metalinguistic training:* The clinician, client, and parent participate in games and activities that present different variations of phonemic introspection, which the parent can use in home practice.
- *Phonetic-production training:* The clinician teaches the client the phonetic components of the phoneme. The parent conducts home practice in both the perception and production of the therapy target or targets.
- *Multiple-exemplar training:* The parent carries out contrastive-production training and conceptual training in a variety of play activities.
- *Homework:* The parent carries out treatment activities in the home as directed by the clinician. The homework supplements the treatment activities completed during the client's previous treatment session.

Research Note	Home practice should be conducted approximately 5 to 6 days per week. Parent and child sessions should be carried out one to three times per day for 5 to 7 minutes.

Bowen and Cupples, 1999, 2004.

The schedule of home intervention activities is similar to that conducted by the clinician, but the activities will be of shorter duration because of time allocation constraints. Furthermore, treatment is provided in 10-week training and vacation blocks. Clients receive direct treatment for approximately 10 weeks and are then dismissed for about 10 weeks. When starting a new training block, a review of the client's phonological status is conducted to plan the current 10-week segment of treatment.

CONCLUSION

This chapter discusses treatments that embody different theoretical perspectives in detail so that clinicians may use them with clients who demonstrate sound system disorders. An exhaustive review by Gierut (1998) identified 64 different treatment studies that were published in the journals of the American Speech-Language-Hearing Association (ASHA) between 1980 and 1995. The author concludes that treatment efficacy was indeed demonstrated across these studies. Dependent variable measures have consistently shown positive changes "in improving speech intelligibility and in bridging the gap between the sound system of the child and that of the target phonology" (Gierut, 1998, p. S89). However, the studies differed as a function of the underlying theories that guided the research, indicating heterogeneity among clients with sound system errors.

A clinician can be confident that a treatment based on one of the tested theories will be of benefit to a client. However, is the selected treatment also the optimum treatment? This is the critical issue in choosing a treatment for a sound system disorder. The selection process mandates that the clinician consider all relevant assessment data and develop a cogent treatment based on a legitimate theoretical rationale. Clinicians must implement the treatment that will maximize the client's learning of phonetic and phonemic concepts. The decision process is one that the clinician, not this author, must make in conjunction with the client's caregivers and client, when appropriate. It must be based on research and state-of-the-art clinical practice. Therefore the clinician must be familiar with the current literature and the application of that literature to the assessment and treatment of clients with sound system disorders.

Treatment of sound system disorders continues to improve as clinicians systematically examine different treatment variables, but a number of abiding issues remain.

ABIDING TREATMENT ISSUES

Phonetic versus Phonemic Errors

Differentiating between phonetic and phonemic errors is not a clear-cut process for the clinician, and readers need to be cognizant of this issue. A number of variables have been proposed in the literature to differentiate between phonetic- and phonemic-based disorders, and these different measures may be used in the diagnostic process. However, the reader should note that some clients demonstrate sound system errors that include both phonetic and phonemic errors. In addition, overlap occurs in the consistency of errors and sound stimulability. That is, both phonetic and phonemic errors may be consistent and nonstimulable (Liles and Williams, 2006; Table 2-4).

Self-Monitoring Tasks

The use of self-monitoring tasks has been included in a number of treatments that are quite diverse in terms of their underlying theory

Table 2-4
Phonetic versus Phonemic Errors

VARIABLE	PHONETIC	PHONEMIC
Number of errors	Few errors	Multiple errors
Sound inventory	Few missing sounds	Many missing sounds
Distributional differences	Sound never used	Sound used in certain positions
Intelligibility	Generally intelligible	Generally unintelligible
Error consistency	Invariable errors	Variable errors
Stimulability	Stimulable	Nonstimulable

(Shriberg and Kwiatkowski, 1987). These self-monitoring techniques include the following (Koegel et al., 1986):

- The client monitors correct and incorrect productions of target sounds in production practice.
- The client may identify, discriminate, or monitor (or a combination of these actions) the production of another person, such as the clinician or caregiver.
- The client assesses the accuracy of his or her productions in more spontaneous treatment activities such as conversational exchanges.

Although definitive data are lacking (Bernthal and Bankson, 2004), preliminary data suggest that self-monitoring is beneficial in promoting generalization. Clinicians should consider the inclusion of self-monitoring in treatment.

Phonological Awareness

Guidelines regarding the use of phonological awareness activities for children with sound system disorders are somewhat variable. Some of the treatments described include phonological awareness as an integral component of the treatment (Bowen and Cupples, 1999; Howell and Dean, 1994). However, Bernhardt (2005) recommends that if deficits in phonological awareness are seen, they should be treated directly if improvement is not demonstrated as the result of treating the client's sound system disorder, which may be unlikely (Gillon, 2000). Tyler (2005b) does not target phonological awareness unless the client is in elementary school and a deficit has been identified through standardized testing. Others such as Justice and Schuele (2004) recommend that awareness activities be incorporated into sound system treatment through the use of activities such as rhyme, alliteration, and other introspective activities. Current thinking indicates that phonological awareness needs to be evaluated via standardized testing if skills are suspect. Phonological-awareness treatment would then be carried out in conjunction with sound system treatment, not independent from sound system treatment (Stackhouse et al., 2002).

Phonemic Perception

Early descriptions of sound system treatment included phonemic perception training; however, most contemporary treatments, with the exception of the work of Rvachew (2005), do not contain such a treatment component (Bernthal and Bankson, 2004). Some researchers believe that perceptual skills are an implicit part of current treatments because the client is being exposed to examples of the target sound through production, self-evaluation of target productions, and phonological awareness. Smit (2004) points out that discrimination tasks can be categorized as internal or external. Internal discrimination is the ability of the client to discriminate between the error sound and the target sound in his or her productions, whereas external discrimination is the ability of the client to discriminate between the error and target sound as produced by another person.

Rvachew and colleagues (2004) conducted a literature review and concluded that many children with sound system errors have phonemic perception deficits. The authors suggest that children's perceptual and production errors are a function of a difference between their underlying phonological knowledge and the adult's system of underlying phonological contrasts. If a child does have a speech sound discrimination problem, then it should be treated. Assessment can be conducted using the Speech Production Perception Task proposed by Locke (1980), which is a measure developed to evaluate a client's perception of his or her sound system errors. This is an external task that is based on the child's error productions contrasted with the target and control sounds. Another previously mentioned assessment tool is SAILS (Avaaz Innovations, 1994). This computerized program contains subsets that target speech sounds frequently misarticulated by young clients. The target sound is embedded in the pre- or postvocalic position of a word, along a perceptual continuum that ranges from correct to incorrect tokens. The program is also used in treatment to assist the client in developing appropriate phonemic categories for the sounds that are in error.

Phonotactics

Phonotactic constraints are the rules of a language that govern permissible word and syllable shapes (Velleman, 1998). Most clinicians target individual sound segments, but some clients require treatment for phonotactic problems. Clinicians need to be cognizant of this when evaluating clients and planning therapy. Velleman (2005) indicates that young clients with severe sound system disorders frequently do not have the necessary syllable and word shapes required for the juxtaposition of newly taught sound segments. For instance, a client may delete all final consonants so that the CVC is not realized; instead the client uses the CV shape. Some target sounds or sound classes may be too difficult for the client until he or she can produce CVC shapes.

Velleman (2002) lists the following phonotactic patterns that are of clinical relevance:
- Deletion of initial consonants
- Deletion of final consonants
- Harmony and reduplication
- Reduction of multisyllabic words
- Reduction or an error of word stress
- Reduction of consonant clusters at the initiation, ending, or middle of a word or syllable

Specific suggestions for treating phonotactic problems can be found in Bernhardt (1994), Velleman (2002), and Chapter 3.

Vowel Errors

Clinicians generally treat consonant errors with little attention to the client's vowel system. Pollock and Berni (2003) studied vowel production in large groups of preschool-aged normal speakers and speakers with sound system disorders. They reported that clients with moderate to severe involvement are at risk for vowel errors. Clinicians should be aware of this and monitor vowel production in clients with moderate to severe sound system disorders. If errors are present, then treatment may be necessary (Gibbon and Beck, 2002). The reader should refer to Chapter 5 for treatment information.

Measurement of Performance

Some treatments specify certain performance criteria that a client must meet, whereas others do not. Measurement of client performance is very important, particularly in the advent of evidence-based management (Baker and McLeod, 2004; Justice and Fey, 2004). Practitioners need to select a treatment that is appropriate and grounded in some degree of scientific rigor, and they must use care when measuring each client's response to the treatment. The measurement of the client's response to training trials and generalization provide objective data to evaluate the effectiveness of a treatment (see Chapter 1). The collection of training trial data enables the clinician to determine whether the client is responding to the treatment and when to change presentation cues and levels of the treatment. For instance, the clinician must set a criterion for the completion of individual training tasks. If the client is producing the target in words after an imitative cue from the clinician, then the clinician establishes a response criterion for completion that is based on some selected time or count measure. In this example, the client must produce the target item imitatively in a list of six practice words or contrasts at an accuracy rate of 80% in two consecutive blocks of 20 training trials. When the client meets the criterion, practice shifts to production of the practice words elicited by pictures alone. In addition to an individual task response criterion, daily accuracy percentages of the sound or contrast should be taken. The training trial criterion tells the clinician when to move ahead with the treatment, and the daily overall percentage of performance furnishes data on the client's inclusive performance to the components of the treatment. The data also inform the clinician when the treatment is not working so that changes in the treatment or a new treatment may be introduced.

The collection of generalization data assists in determining the amount of learning outside of therapy, which is the ultimate goal of treatment (Baker and McLeod, 2004). That is, treatment is designed to foster generalization because teaching every example of a target or target contrast is impossible. The measurement of generalization discussed in Chapter 1 is a critical adjunct to any treatment program. The acid test of a treatment is generalization to untaught items, untaught sounds, and sound classes that are related and various situational contexts. Similar to client performance data, identification of lack of generalization is also important. For instance, Elbert and colleagues (1990) recommend that the number of words used in treatment be increased if generalization is lacking. Additional suggestions for facilitating generalization can be found in Bernthal and Bankson (2004).

Dismissal Criteria

Most treatment programs do not set dismissal criteria; instead the clinician must measure performance and decide whether dismissal is warranted. An investigation by Diedrich and Bangert (1980) examined the performance of school-aged clients with /r/ or /s/ residual errors who received treatment from a number of different clinicians. The researchers found that clients who achieved 75% level of accuracy on conversational probes could be dismissed from treatment. Williams (2003) developed the multiple oppositions approach for preschool clients with moderate to severe phonological disorders. The author indicates that treatment is terminated for a specific phoneme collapse when the client achieves 50% accuracy or higher on a conversational probe.

McKercher and colleagues (1995) examined the performance of seven clients with mild to severe speech sound disorders. Clients were taught by a number of different experimental treatments, and generalization was assessed with a 15-item picture assessment task that contained the target sound in the prevocalic, postvocalic, and intervocalic word positions. The task was administered pretreatment, posttreatment, and 6 to 8 weeks after the termination of treatment. The results of their study indicate that clients who achieve an accuracy level of 75% at posttreatment maintain or improve their performance on target sounds after the withdrawal of treatment. These findings show that generalization measurement is an important adjunct to treatment, and a performance level of 75% for either conversation or word probes should be considered when deciding to dismiss a client or introduce a new treatment goal. In either case, periodic probes should be taken, including after dismissal to monitor retention or regression.

Caregivers in the Intervention Process

The client's caregivers (including parents, teachers, and siblings) can play an important role in treatment, provided they are willing to participate in the process (Figure 2-4). Moreover, the NOMS shows that more substantial gains in treatment of sound system disorders are associated with caregiver participation in treatment. Caregivers can assume passive or active roles in treatment, or they can assume both (Bowen and Cupples, 1999, 2004). The passive role is one of understanding the nature of the problem, discussing the treatment to be introduced, asking questions, being the recipient of periodic progress reports, establishing a bond with the clinician, and promoting a positive attitude to the child regarding treatment. The caregiver may also provide verbal feedback to the clinician, answer satisfaction surveys (Rvachew and Nowak, 2001), or complete informational questionnaires (Tyler and Tolbert, 2002).

An active role is one of participation in the intervention process and should be implemented only if the caregiver expresses a willingness

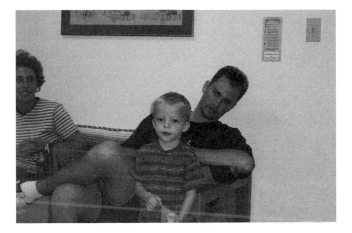

***Figure* 2-4** ■ Client's caregivers play an important role in the treatment of sound system disorders.

to do so and is trained appropriately. A caregiver program, if done properly, can enhance the treatment process by providing increased opportunities for response in a positive environment. If a clinician wishes to implement a parent program, then the program developed by Bowen and Cupples (1999, 2004) can be used, or it can be adapted to fit the needs of the client and clinician. The roles of the participants are clearly delineated, and recent data reported by Bowen and Cupples (2004) suggest that the Parents and Children Together (PACT) treatment program is an effective intervention for children with sound system disorders.

Scheduling Treatment Sessions

Little data are available on this topic. Bernthal and Bankson (2004) reviewed the literature and made the following recommendations:

- Distributed practice appears superior to massed practice. That is, treating the client in three 20-minute sessions per week is better than having one 60-minute session per week.
- For some clients, block scheduling (in which clients are scheduled four to five times per week for a period of 8 to 10 weeks) may be superior to long-term scheduling of one to two sessions per week across a greater time span.
- Clients with severe sound system disorders need ongoing services; consequently, long-term treatment rather than block scheduling may be more beneficial.

Bowen and Cupples (1999, 2004) formulated a comprehensive treatment approach that uses 10-week blocks of treatment. They reasoned that block scheduling allows the child to acquire his or her phonology on a gradual basis. Clients receive treatment for 10 weeks from the clinician, and they also receive parent-administered treatment; the program is then withdrawn for 10 weeks. During the withdrawal period, parents are encouraged to engage in informal production and metalinguistic tasks with the child. Preliminary data suggest that the treatment is effective with preschool children with moderate to severe sound system disorders.

Use of Technology

Developments in computer technology allow clinicians to incorporate the technology into their management of persons with communication disorders at a relatively low cost (McGuire, 1995). In a review of computer applications for clients with sound system disorders, Gierut (1998) indicated that computer applications are a useful component in treatment. Early treatment activities may need to be clinician directed in cases involving clients acquiring correct target productions when models are needed, as well as cases involving young children who might be easily distracted in treatment. Computer instruction can be used effectively after the client has acquired the specific contrast or sound and is ready to integrate the target in his or her phonological system. Masterson and Rvachew (1999) discussed additional information regarding the implementation of computer hardware and software in the treatment of sound system disorders.

Oral Motor Treatment

Oral motor treatment (OMT) is different from phonetic or phonemic treatments because it targets nonspeech motor movements and oral postures with the aim of developing motor patterns required for speech sound production, for strengthening the muscles used in speech production, or both (Strode and Chamberlain, 1997). Various nonspeech exercise movements, instruments such as horns and whistles, and stimulatory techniques are used as facilitating agents before or concurrent with treatment for sound system disorders (Marshalla, 2001). The preponderance of research supports direct treatment (not OMT) as an effective change agent for children with sound system disorders (Bowen, 2005; Forrest, 2002; Gierut, 1998; Guisti Braislin and Cascella, 2005; Weismer, 1997, 2006).

SUMMARY

This chapter provides a detailed discussion of contemporary treatments derived from different theoretical rationales. Clinicians use these treatments to remediate sound system disorders in clients with no known structural, sensory, or neurological deficits. Intervention data suggest that the treatments are effective in modifying sound system disorders. The reader should keep in mind that the clinician has the key role of assessing the client's disorder and selecting the appropriate treatment for the child. One specific treatment is not sufficient for all clients with sound system disorders. In conclusion, Shriberg and Kwiatkowski (1982) state the following:

> Management programs that focus only on content may fail to account for critical client-clinician factors in the affective domain. As in all areas in education, the task is to create an optimum balance between an environment favorable to learning, and efficient delivery of the technical elements of that which is to be learned.

REFERENCES

Avaaz Innovations: *SAILS: Speech Assessment and Interactive Learning System*, version 1.2 [computer software], London, Ontario, Canada, 1994, Author.

Baker E, McLeod S: Evidence-based management of phonological impairment in children, *Chil Lang Teach Ther* 20:261-285, 2004.

Barlow JA, Gierut JA: Minimal pair approaches to phonological remediation, *Semin Speech Lang* 23:57-67, 2002.

Bauman-Waengler J: *Articulatory and phonological impairments*, ed 2, Boston, 2004, Allyn & Bacon.

Bernhardt B: Phonological intervention techniques for syllable and word structure development, *Clin Commun Disord* 4:54-65, 1994.

Bernhardt B: Selection of phonological goals and targets: not just an exercise in phonological analysis. In Kamhi AG, Pollock KE, editors: *Phonological disorders in children*, Baltimore, 2005, Paul H Brookes.

Bernthal JE, Bankson NW: *Articulation and phonological disorders*, ed 5, Boston, 2004, Allyn & Bacon.

Bowen C: *Developmental phonological disorders: a practical guide for families and teachers*, Melbourne, Australia, 1998, The Australian Council for Educational Research.

Bowen C: What is the evidence for oral motor therapy? Acquiring knowledge in speech, language and hearing, *Speech Pathol Aus* October:144-147, 2005.

Bowen C, Cupples L: Parents and children together (PACT): a collaborative approach to phonological therapy, *Int J Lang Commun Disord* 34:35-55, 1999.

Bowen C, Cupples L: The role of families in optimizing phonological therapy outcomes, *Child Lang Teach Ther* 20:245-260, 2004.

Camarata S: The application of naturalistic conversation training to speech production in children with speech disabilities, *J Appl Behav Anal* 26:173-182, 1993.

Davis BL: Clinical diagnosis of developmental speech disorders. In Kamhi AG, Pollock KE, editors: *Phonological disorders in children*, Baltimore, 2005, Paul H Brookes.

Dean EC, Howell J, Waters D et al: A metalinguistic approach to the treatment of phonological disorder in children, *Clin Linguist Phon* 9:1-19, 1995.

Diedrich WM, Bangert J: *Articulation learning*, Houston, 1980, College-Hill Press.

Elbert M, Dinnesen DA, Swartzlander P et al: Generalization to conversational speech, *J Speech Hear Disord* 55:694-699, 1990.

Elbert M, Gierut J: *Handbook of clinical phonology*, San Diego, 1986, College-Hill Press.

Elbert M, Shelton RL, Arndt WB: A task for the evaluation of articulation change. I. Development of methodology, *J Speech Hear Disord* 44:459-471, 1967.

Fey ME: *Language intervention with young children*, Boston, 1986, Allyn & Bacon.

Forrest K: Are oral-motor exercises useful in the treatment of phonological/articulatory disorders? *Semin Speech Lang* 23:15-25, 2002.

Gibbon FE, Beck JM: Therapy for abnormal vowels in children with phonological impairment. In Ball MJ, Gibbon FE, editors: *Vowel disorders*, Woburn, Mass, 2002, Butterworth-Heinemann.

Gierut JA: Maximal opposition approach to phonological treatment, *J Speech Hear Disord* 54:9-19, 1989.

Gierut JA: Differential learning of phonological oppositions, *J Speech Hear Res* 33:540-549, 1990.

Gierut JA: Treatment efficacy; functional phonological disorders in children, *J Speech Hear Res* 41(suppl):S85-S100, 1998.

Gierut JA: Complexity in phonological treatment: clinical factors, *Lang Speech Hear Serv Sch* 32:229-241, 2001.

Gierut JA: Phonological intervention. In Kamhi AG, Pollock KE, editors: *Phonological disorders in children*, Baltimore, 2005, Paul H Brookes.

Gillon GT: The efficacy of phonological awareness intervention for children with spoken language impairment, *Lang Speech Hear Serv Sch* 31:126-141, 2000.

Griffiths J, Miner L: *Phonetic context drillbook*, Englewood Cliffs, NJ, 1979, Prentice-Hall.

Guisti Braislin MA, Cascella PW: A preliminary investigation of the efficacy of oral motor exercises for children with mild articulation disorders, *Int J Rehabil Res* 28:263-266, 2005.

Hodson BW: Phonological remediation: a cycles approach. In Creaghead NA, Newman PW, Secord WA, editors: *Assessment and remediation of articulatory and phonological disorders,* Columbus, Ohio, 1989, Merrill.

Hodson B, Paden D: *Targeting intelligible speech: a phonological approach to remediation,* San Diego, 1983, College-Hill Press.

Hoffman PR: Synergistic development of phonetic skills, *Lang Speech Hear Serv Sch* 23:254-260, 1992.

Hoffman PR, Norris JA: Manipulating complex input to promote self-organization of a neuro-network. In Kamhi AG, Pollock KE, editors: *Phonological disorders in children,* Baltimore, 2005, Paul H Brookes.

Hoffman PR, Norris JA, Monjure J: Comparison of process targeting and whole language treatments for phonologically delayed preschool children, *Lang Speech Hear Serv Sch* 21:102-109, 1990.

Hoffman PR, Schuckers GH, Daniloff RG: *Children's phonetic disorders,* Boston, 1989, College-Hill Press.

Howell J, Dean EC: *Treating phonological disorders in children: metaphon-theory to practice,* ed 2, London, 1994, Whurr.

Justice LM, Fey ME: Evidence-based practice in schools, *ASHA Leader* 21:4-5, 30-32, September 2004.

Justice LM, Schuele CM: Phonological awareness: description, assessment, and intervention. In Bernthal JE, Bankson NW, editors: *Articulation and phonological disorders,* ed 5, Boston, 2004, Allyn & Bacon.

Kamhi AG: Summary, reflections, and future directions. In Kamhi AG, Pollock KE, editors: *Phonological disorders in children,* Baltimore, 2005, Paul H Brookes.

Kent RD: Contextual facilitation of correct sound production, *Lang Speech Hear Serv Sch* 13:66-76, 1982.

Klein ES: Phonological/traditional approaches to articulation therapy: a retrospective group comparison, *Lang Speech Hear Serv Sch* 27:314-323, 1996.

Koegel LK, Koegel RL, Ingham JC: Programming rapid generalization of correct articulation through self-monitoring procedures, *J Speech Hear Disord* 51:24-32, 1986.

Kucera H, Francis WN: *Computational analysis of present-day American English,* Providence, RI, 1967, Brown University.

Liles T, Williams AL: *A multiple oppositions approach with a mixed phonetic/phonemic disorder.* Paper presented at the annual convention of the American Speech-Language-Hearing Association, Miami, November 2006.

Locke J: The inference of speech perception in the phonologically disordered child. II. Some clinically novel procedures, their use, some findings, *J Speech Hear Disord* 45:445-468, 1980.

Lowe RJ: *Phonology: assessment and intervention applications in speech pathology,* Philadelphia, 1994, Williams & Wilkins.

Manning WH, Keappock NE, Stick SL: The use of auditory masking to estimate automatization of correct articulatory production, *J Speech Hear Disord* 41:143-149, 1976.

Marshalla P: *Oral motor techniques in articulation and phonological therapy,* Kirkland, Wash, 2001, Marshalla Speech & Language Service.

Masterson JJ, Rvachew S: Use of technology in phonology intervention, *Semin Speech Lang* 20:233-250, 1999.

McCauley RJ, Skenes LL: Contrastive stress, phonetic context, and misarticulations of /r/ in young speakers, *J Speech Hear Res* 30:114-121, 1987.

McDonald ET: *Articulation testing and treatment: a sensory motor approach,* Pittsburgh, 1964, Stanwix House.

McGuire RA: Computer-based instrumentation: issues in clinical application, *Lang Speech Hear Serv Sch* 26:223-231, 1995.

McKercher M, McFarlane L, Schneider P: Phonological treatment dismissal: optimal criteria, *J Speech Lang Pathol Audiol* 19:115-123, 1995.

Miccio AW: A treatment program for enhancing stimulability. In Kamhi AG, Pollock KE, editors: *Phonological disorders in children,* Baltimore, 2005, Paul H Brookes.

Morrisette ML, Gierut JA: Lexical organization and phonological change in treatment, *J Speech Lang Hear Res* 45:143-159, 2002.

Netsell R: Construction and use of a bite-block for the evaluation and treatment of speech disorders, *J Speech Hear Disord* 50:100-109, 1985.

Norris JA, Hoffman PR: Language intervention within naturalistic environments, *Lang Speech Hear Serv Sch* 21:72-84, 1990.

Norris JA, Hoffman PR: Goals and targets: facilitating the self-organizing nature of a neuro-network. In Kamhi AG, Pollock KE, editors: *Phonological disorders in children,* Baltimore, 2005, Paul H Brookes.

Paul R: *Language disorders from infancy through adolescence,* ed 3, St Louis, 2007, Mosby.

Pollock KE, Berni MC: Incidence of non-rhotic vowel errors in children: data from the Memphis Vowel Project, *Clin Linguist Phon* 17:393-401, 2003.

Ruscello DM: A motor skill learning treatment program for sound system disorders, *Semin Speech Lang* 14:106-118, 1993.

Rvachew S: Speech perception training can facilitate sound production learning, *J Speech Hear Res* 37:347-357, 1994.

Rvachew S: The importance of phonetic factors in phonological intervention. In Kamhi AG, Pollock KE, editors: *Phonological disorders in children,* Baltimore, 2005, Paul H Brookes.

Rvachew S, Jamieson D: Perception of voiceless fricatives by children with a functional articulation disorder, *J Speech Hear Disord* 54:193-208, 1989.

Rvachew S, Nowak N: The effect of target selection strategy on phonological learning, *J Speech Lang Hear Res* 44:610-623, 2001.

Rvachew S, Nowak N, Cloutier G: Effect of phonemic perception training on the speech production and phonological awareness skills of children with expressive phonological delay, *Am J Speech Lang Pathol* 13:250-263, 2004.

Rvachew S, Rafaat S, Martin M: Stimulability, speech perception skills, and the treatment of phonological disorders, *Am J Speech Lang Pathol* 8:33-43, 1999.

Saben CB, Ingham JC: The effects of minimal pairs treatment on the speech sound production of two children with phonologic disorders, *J Speech Lang Hear Res* 34:1023-1040: 1991.

Schmidt RA, Wrisberg CA: *Motor learning and performance*, ed 2, Champaign, Ill, 2000, Human Kinetics.

Secord W: *Eliciting sounds: techniques for clinicians*, San Antonio, 1981a, Psychological Corporation.

Secord W: *C-PAC: clinical probes of articulation consistency*, San Antonio, 1981b, Psychological Corporation.

Secord W: The traditional approach to treatment. In Creaghead NA, Newman PW, Secord WA, editors: *Assessment and remediation of articulatory and phonological disorders*, ed 2, Columbus, Ohio, 1989, Merrill.

Secord W, Shine RE: *Target words for contextual training*, Sedona, Ariz, 1997, Red Rock Educational Publications.

Shine RE: Articulatory production training: a sensory-motor approach. In Creaghead NA, Newman PW, Secord WA, editors: *Assessment and remediation of articulatory and phonological disorders*, ed 2, Columbus, Ohio, 1989, Merrill.

Shriberg LD: A response evocation program for /ɝ/, *J Speech Hear Disord* 40:92-105, 1975.

Shriberg L, Kwiatkowski J: Phonological disorders. II. A conceptual framework for management, *J Speech Hear Disord* 47:242-255, 1982.

Shriberg L, Kwiatkowski J: A retrospective study of spontaneous generalization in speech-delayed children, *Lang Speech Hear Serv Sch* 18:144-157, 1987.

Sloat C, Taylor CH, Hoard JE: *Introduction to phonology*, Englewood Cliffs, NJ, 1978, Prentice-Hall.

Skelton SL: Concurrent task sequencing in single-phoneme phonologic treatment and generalization, *J Commun Disord* 37:131-156, 2004.

Smit AB: *Articulation and phonology resource guide for school-age children and adults*, Clifton Park, NY, 2004, Thomson Delmar Learning.

Stackhouse J, Wells B, Pascoe M et al: From phonological therapy to phonological awareness, *Semin Speech Lang* 23:27-42, 2002.

Strode R, Chamberlain C: *Easy does it for articulation: an oral-motor approach*, East Moline, Ill, 1997, Lingui Systems.

Tyler AA: Language-based intervention for phonological disorders, *Semin Speech Lang* 23:69-81, 2002.

Tyler AA: Assessment for determining a communication profile. In Kamhi AG, Pollock KE, editors: *Phonological disorders in children*, Baltimore, 2005a, Paul H Brookes.

Tyler AA: Planning and monitoring intervention programs. In Kamhi AG, Pollock KE, editors: *Phonological disorders in children*, Baltimore, 2005b, Paul H Brookes.

Tyler AA, Edwards ML, Saxman JH: Clinical application of two phonologically-based treatment procedures, *J Speech Hear Disord* 52:393-409, 1987.

Tyler AA, Lewis KE, Haskill A et al: Efficacy and cross domain effects of a morphosyntax and phonology intervention, *Lang Speech Hear Serv Sch* 33:52-66, 2002.

Tyler AA, Tolbert LC: Speech-language assessment in the clinical setting, *Am J Speech Lang Pathol* 8:33-43, 2002.

Velleman SL: *Making phonology functional,* Woburn, Mass, 1998, Butterworth-Heinemann.

Velleman SL: Phonotactic therapy, *Semin Speech Lang* 23:43-53, 2002.

Velleman SL: Special considerations in intervention. In Kamhi AG, Pollock KE, editors: *Phonological disorders in children*, Baltimore, 2005, Paul H Brookes.

Weiner F: Treatment of phonological disability using the method of meaningful minimal contrast: two case studies, *J Speech Hear Disord* 46:97-103, 1981.

Weismer G: *Assessment of oromotor, nonspeech gestures in speech-language pathology: a critical review,* Tucson, Ariz, 1997, National Center for Neurogenic Communication Disorders at the University of Arizona (videotape).

Weismer G: Philosophy of research in motor speech disorders, *Clin Linguist Phon* 20:315-349, 2006.

Williams AL: *Speech disorders resource guide for preschool children,* Clifton Park, NJ, 2003, Thomson Delmar Learning.

Williams AL: A model and structure for phonological intervention. In Kamhi AG, Pollock KE, editors: *Phonological disorders in children*, Baltimore, 2005, Paul H Brookes.

Williams AL: *Sound contrasts in phonology (SCIP),* Eau Claire, Wis, 2006, Thinking Publications (CD-ROM).

Wingo JW, Hoshiko M: Differential effectiveness of six information-input procedures utilized to teach unfamiliar sounds in isolation, *J Speech Hear Res* 15:256-263, 1972.

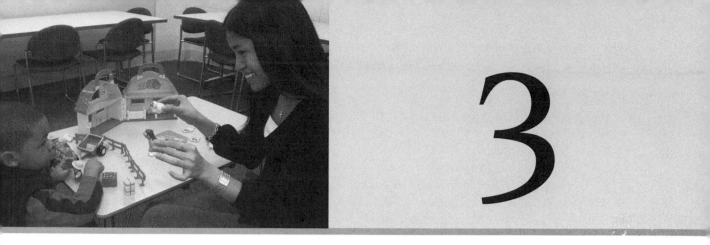

3

Treatment of Children with Developmental Motor Speech Disorders

LEARNING GOALS
- Identify the five distinct levels of output processing as introduced by Caruso and Strand.
- Define childhood apraxia of speech (CAS), and list the diagnostic variables associated with this disorder.
- Define developmental dysarthria and discuss its various manifestations.
- Compare and contrast CAS and developmental dysarthria.
- List several general treatment recommendations for CAS, and briefly describe integral stimulation.
- Outline the systems approach to the treatment of developmental dysarthria.

Developmental motor speech disorders are neurophysiologically based disorders that involve either the planning and programming or the execution of movement during speech. These particular disorders typically have an onset during early childhood as the result of a congenital problem or may be acquired later in development as the result of illness or injury. **Childhood apraxia of speech (CAS)** is a deficit in planning and programming of skilled movement, whereas **dysarthria** is an execution problem with skilled movement.

THEORETICAL MODEL AND DEFINITIONS

Caruso and Strand (1999) have proposed a model of speech production that posits five distinct levels of output processing. Accordingly, the generation of a speech message begins at the cognitive or ideational level where the communicative message originates or is conceived and proceeds to the second or linguistic level. At the linguistic level, lexical access, phonological patterning, and word order framing interact to create a linguistic version of the message. At the third level of processing, the linguistic message is converted into actual speech units through processes that occur at the sensorimotor planning stage. The goal is to produce an acoustic output that can be perceived and comprehended by a listener. After the planning stage or third level of output processing, articulatory temporal and positioning variables are coded at the sensorimotor programming level. The authors indicate that movement coordination must be very specific, yet very flexible, to meet all of the production demands that must be accounted for in speech production. The final stage of the process is one of sensorimotor execution. At this final processing stage, the message is transmitted to the listener. The reader should note that planning (Output Level III), programming

(Output Level IV), and execution (Output Level V) involve both motor and sensory components. That is, movement is a motor function, but sensory information plays an important role in the creation of messages that are produced for different listeners.

The proposed model of speech production introduces five levels of output processing: (1) cognitive and ideational level, (2) linguistic level, (3) planning level, (4) programming level, and (5) execution level.	*Research* Note

Caruso and Strand, 1999.

The description of Caruso and Stand's model is an oversimplification, but it provides a starting point to conceptualize motor speech disorders. According to the model, CAS is a developmental motor speech disorder that occurs at the level of sensorimotor planning, whereas developmental dysarthria is a motor speech disorder of sensorimotor execution. The authors hypothesize that children with CAS experience difficulty in formulating or planning speech; however, at this time researchers do not know what constitutes the basic planning unit of speech. Some speech scientists believe that the syllable is the basic unit; however, this has not been established. Whatever the unit, these clients need intervention to assist in acquiring appropriate motor plans for speech production.

After being planned and programmed, the movement sequence is realized through execution. Clients with developmental dysarthria exhibit difficulties in the execution of articulatory movements and possibly other components of speech production because of central or peripheral nervous system damage. Although Caruso and Strand (1999) have proposed a theoretical model of speech production that attempts to explain the neurophysiology of developmental motor speech disorders, this theory has not been proved or disproved. The reader needs to be mindful of the fact that other theories have been offered to explain normal physiology (Kent, 1999) and developmental motor speech disorders (Love, 1992; Robin, 1992). Theory development and testing is very important in attempting to understand a disorder and formulating appropriate ways to assess and treat it.

CHILDHOOD APRAXIA OF SPEECH

The Ad Hoc Committee on Apraxia of Speech in Children (American Speech-Language-Hearing Association, 2006) conducted an extensive review of the literature and formulated the following draft definition of CAS that includes a proposed cause, core deficits, and effects of the disorder on communication and literacy development:

> Childhood apraxia of speech (CAS) is a subtype of severe childhood speech sound disorder due to unidentified neurological differences likely of genetic origin. The core deficits arise at linguistic or early speech motor processing levels. Symptomatology, which changes with age, may include age-inappropriate vowel/diphthong errors, unusual and variable errors in repeated attempts at words, increased number and severity of errors with increasing word and utterance length, and prosodic disturbances. CAS places a child at increased risk for persisting problems in speech, language, and literacy.

Clients with CAS generally have intellectual skills that are within normal limits and no oral structural deficits that might interfere with speech production (Davis and Velleman, 2000). Sensory mechanisms such as vision, hearing, tactile, and kinesthetic sensation are also normal. Clients with CAS often show a gap between receptive and expressive language, with receptive skills normal or near normal and expressive skills below levels of normative expectation. CAS clients are also at risk for persisting language problems, and they may experience difficulties in the acquisition of reading and spelling (Lewis et al., 2004).

Research Note	Most clients with CAS have normal intellectual skills and no oral structural deficits to interfere with speech production; however, they generally have a coexisting language disorder.

Davis and Velleman, 2000.

Shriberg and colleagues (1997) estimate the prevalence of CAS at approximately one to two clients per thousand; however, the diagnosis of CAS appears to be assigned to clients on a more frequent basis (Davis and Velleman, 2000). This discrepancy may be in large part because of the variability in diagnostic criteria for CAS and third-party reimbursement issues. Although CAS remains an elusive diagnostic entity (Forrest, 2002), clients showing such disorders require treatment. What segmental, phonotactic, prosodic, speech motor, and oral motor variables might be associated with CAS? The work of Davis and associates (Davis et al., 1998; Davis and Velleman, 2000) has helped clinicians understand the different problems exhibited by clients with CAS.

The variables associated with CAS are listed in Box 3-1. The variables with asterisks contrast CAS characteristics with characteristics of severe sound system disorder. That is, the items with asterisks are more likely associated with CAS than with severe sound system disorder. However, not all clients will show all of the symptoms; instead, clusters of the listed symptoms may be present in their speech. In addition, some features occur infrequently. For instance, **hypernasality,** which is a resonance disorder, is sometimes identified as a feature in the speech of some clients with CAS. Generally, clients with possible CAS have very limited consonant and vowel inventories. In addition, many of their production errors consist of sound deletions that may affect syllable composition, and they exhibit vowel placement errors. Clients also show variability in the repetition of words and word sequences, and production errors often increase in relation to grammatical complexity. Another behavior reported for some clients is **groping.** This type of rehearsal behavior appears as a means for the client to explore different articulatory positions in an effort to achieve the correct articulatory placement for a sound. Clients may also have difficulty with imitative speech skills and lack prosodic variation in their production of words, phrases, and sentences. Finally, **diadochokinetic tasks** are frequently difficult for

---

BOX 3-1   *Diagnostic Variables Associated with Childhood Apraxia of Speech*

Segmental, Phonotactic, and Prosodic Variables
Restricted consonant and vowel phonetic inventories
Primary use of simple syllable shapes
Frequent deletion errors
High frequency of vowel errors*
Variable performance in the production of words and word sequences*
Increase in production errors with an increase in linguistic complexity*
Groping or rehearsal postures present*
Difficulty with imitation*
Lack of prosodic variation*

Speech Motor Control Variable
Deficient diadochokinesis*

Oral Motor Variable
Problems with producing nonspeech oral motor movements*

*Reported as major features of childhood apraxia of speech.

CAS clients, and some are reported to experience problems in producing isolated and sequential nonspeech oral movements.

DEVELOPMENTAL DYSARTHRIA

Hodge and Wellman (1999) indicate that **developmental dysarthria** is a collective diagnostic term that defines a group of speech disorders resulting from interruption or injury to the developing central or peripheral nervous systems (or injury to both). That is, developmental dysarthria is a movement impairment that interferes with the articulatory production of speech, but it can also include involvement of respiration, phonation, resonation, and prosody (Figure 3-1). Love (1992) indicates that movement disorders of developmental dysarthria may manifest in "disturbances of strength, speed, steadiness, coordination, precision, tone, and range of movement in the speech musculature." Language and literacy development are also concerns because structure, content, and use of language are also emerging during the developmental period.

The different developmental dysarthrias can be identified as a function of the site of neurologic injury, characteristics of neuromuscular damage present in the muscles of speech, and the effects of those characteristics on speech production (Duffy, 2005; Hodge and Wellman, 1999; Love, 1992). **Flaccid dysarthria** is the result of injury to the lower

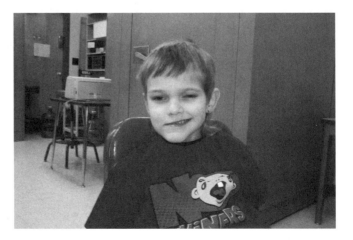

Figure 3-1 ■ A young client with developmental dysarthria shows a right facial weakness. Note that the lip pulls to the unaffected left side when he is asked to smile.

motor neurons located in the brainstem and spinal cord that innervate the speech musculature, their companion cranial and spinal nerves, or the actual muscle fibers that are innervated by the nerves. **Spastic dysarthria** is seen when injury occurs to the upper motor neuron system. The upper motor neuron system includes cortical motor areas and associative areas that are direct or indirect pathways for connection with lower motor neurons located in the brainstem and spinal cord. **Dyskinetic dysarthria** is the result of injury to the basal ganglia, a group of nuclei located at the base of the cerebral hemispheres. The **basal ganglia** (also known as the *extrapyramidal system*) serve an important role in the initiation and control of movement. **Ataxic dysarthria** results from lesions of the cerebellar connections that link with the cortex. The cerebellum is an important component in motor control because it assists in the maintenance of muscle tone and coordinated movement (Figure 3-2). Finally, the client can experience **mixed dysarthrias,** which reflect diffuse damage of the motor system. Each of the dysarthrias has clusters

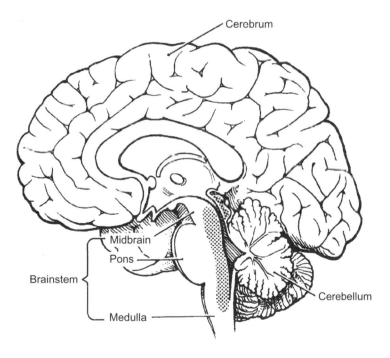

Figure 3-2 ▪ Medial view of the right cerebrum, brainstem, and cerebellum. (From Love RJ, Webb WG: *Neurology for the speech-language pathologist,* ed 4, Boston, 2001, Butterworth-Heinemann.)

BOX 3-2 *Types of Developmental Dysarthria*

Flaccid dysarthria: Damage to lower motor neurons, their cranial and spinal nerves, or the muscle fibers that innervate them
Spastic dysarthria: Damage to upper motor neuron system
Dyskinetic dysarthria: Damage to the basal ganglia
Ataxic dysarthria: Lesions of the cerebellar connections that link with the cortex
Mixed dysarthrias: Diffuse damage of the cerebral motor system

---

of different symptoms that may include impairments of respiration, phonation, resonation, articulation, and prosody (Box 3-2).

In addition to the speech and prosody variables, the practitioner needs to be cognizant of the fact that the neuromuscular impairment also extends to nonspeech oral motor behaviors (Love, 1992). For instance, nonspeech activities such as feeding, swallowing, and saliva control may be impaired to some degree. Postural conditions and mouth breathing can also interfere with dentition, occlusion, and craniofacial growth. In some cases, structural differences that result from neuromuscular impairment may be responsible for the presence of obligatory sound system errors. For example, a client with a neuromuscular impairment also may demonstrate an occlusal problem such as an open bite, and the resulting problem might further prevent production of bilabial sounds because of the accumulating effect of both structure and function.

Research Note | The clinician must be cognizant not only of the speech and prosody variables in clients with developmental dysarthria, but also that the neuromuscular impairment extends to nonspeech oral motor behaviors such as feeding and swallowing.

Love, 1992.

CHILDHOOD APRAXIA OF SPEECH VERSUS DEVELOPMENTAL DYSARTHRIA

Hayden (1994) indicates that CAS and developmental dysarthria are often confused in diagnosis. Consequently, the practitioner should carefully examine the diagnostic features that have been identified.

Robin (1998) provides a succinct summary of features that the practitioner may consider when trying to differentiate CAS from developmental dysarthria (Table 3-1):

1. No paralysis, paresis, ataxia, or involuntary movements occur in CAS such as those found in association with developmental dysarthria.
2. The components of CAS are primarily articulatory and prosodic, whereas dysarthria may include components that affect all speech production subsystems.

Table 3-1
Comparison of Features of Childhood Apraxia of Speech and Developmental Dysarthria

CHARACTERISTIC	CAS	DEVELOPMENTAL DYSARTHRIA
Motor function	Not an associated feature	Associated paralysis, paresis, ataxia, and involuntary movements
Components of the disorder	Primarily articulatory and prosodic	May have components that affect all speech subsystems
Speech production errors	Variable and inconsistent	Consistent and frequently classified as *distortions of the intended target sounds*
Differences according to type of speech	Automatic and purposeful speech may differ	No differences in type of speech
Production errors	Often vary as a function of grammatical complexity	Not a reported feature
Groping	Reported feature	Not a reported feature

CAS, Childhood apraxia of speech.

3. In CAS, speech errors are variable and often inconsistent; however, the errors of developmental dysarthria are generally consistent and frequently classified as *distortions of the intended target sounds*.
4. The client with CAS may exhibit differences between automatic and purposeful speech, but no difference exists between conditions with the developmental dysarthria client.
5. CAS production errors often vary as a function of grammatical complexity, whereas developmental dysarthria errors do not vary in this way.
6. Groping behavior appears to be associated with CAS but not with dysarthria.

TREATMENT OF CHILDHOOD APRAXIA OF SPEECH

A very limited amount of empirical research has examined treatment efficacy for clients with possible CAS (Bahr et al., 1999; McCauley, 2002; Strand and Debertine, 2000). Current treatment concepts are based largely on single-subject case study reports and the expert opinion of professionals who deal with such clients. Although different theoretical rationales have been proposed (Hall, 2000), the general approach to treating CAS is from the perspective of motor skill learning. The principles of this theoretical treatment are incorporated in the phonetic approach (discussed in Chapters 1 and 2). However, one must be mindful of the fact that some young clients have severe problems, and the goal of treatment must shift from a primary emphasis on speech development to communication development. That is, some clients may not be able to acquire productive speech that is intelligible; consequently, some form of augmentative or alternative communication may be needed (in combination with speech or exclusively) to facilitate communication. The clinician must measure performance very carefully so that decisions regarding a reasonable expectation for speech and overall communication are formulated. Although the expectation for the client may change, this change needs to be based on objective measurement data collected by the clinician. This same treatment philosophy is also appropriate in the management of young clients who have developmental dysarthria (discussed later).

General Treatment Recommendations

Reports on treatment for CAS indicate that therapy is intensive and generally required over a number of years (Campbell, 1999). The following general intervention recommendations have been proposed by a number of investigators (Bernhardt, 1994; Cumley and Swanson, 1999;

Davis and Velleman, 2000; Hall et al., 2003; Love, 1992; Marquardt and Sussman, 1991; Robin, 1998; Square, 1994; Strand and Debertine, 2000; Strand and Skinder, 1999; Velleman, 1994, 1998, 2003; Velleman and Strand, 1994). As previously mentioned, the treatment recommendations have not been subject to rigorous empirical examination but are based on judicious clinical judgment and a modicum of treatment efficacy research. The recommendations are as follows (Box 3-3):

- The major guiding principle of treatment is to meet the communication needs of the client through *continuous immersion in a variety of communicative interactions.* For some clients on the severe end of the speech production continuum, it may be necessary to implement some form of augmentative and/or alternative communication exclusively or in combination with speech. Caregivers play a vital role; therefore they should acknowledge and reinforce the communicative attempts of the client, whether those attempts are vocalizations or

---

BOX 3-3 *Summary of General CAS Treatment Recommendations*

- The major guiding principle of treatment is to meet the client's needs through continuous immersion in a variety of communicative interactions.
- A motor-skill learning approach is recommended (as opposed to a phonemic approach) to emphasize practice at various levels of linguistic complexity.
- The clinician must be aware of any coexisting communication problems and the need for possible therapeutic intervention.
- The clinician should carry out the treatment frequently.
- Home practice is an important part of treatment.
- In most cases the primary aim of therapy is to attain intelligibility, not completely normal speech.
- The clinician should emphasize metaphonological analysis and self-monitoring.
- The clinician should limit the number of training stimuli.
- Multisensory stimulation may be useful to the client.
- The clinician should consider phonotactics when developing treatment stimuli.
- If the client has a coexisting oral apraxia, then treatment may be introduced to develop nonspeech isolated and sequential oral movements.

CAS, Childhood apraxia of speech.

some form of idiosyncratic gesture in combination with vocalization. The clinician should encourage vocalizations that can be carried out in the context of body movement or activity. For instance, a client can pair vocalization with play. The clinician and client might play with a favorite toy such as a car and make a *vroom* sound while playing. Caregivers also need to provide appropriate models of communication for the client. Idiosyncratic signs or gestures can be modified to more general signs or gestures, and caregivers can model appropriate word targets of the client's vocalizations.

- When the child begins to produce vocalizations consistently, treatment should shift to sounds combined in various syllabic structures. Early-developing consonants such as /b, m, w, m, n, j/ are potential targets. They can be paired with early-developing vowels such as /ɪ, e, æ, ʌ, ɑ/. Potential syllabic configurations may include CV, CVCV, and CVC. The clinician should introduce other consonant sound additions in syllabic shapes that the child uses, and he or she should introduce new syllable shapes with consonants that are in the client's inventory. The clinician should vary practice with syllables to allow for motor planning; consequently, activities such as rehearsal matrices (summarized in Chapter 2) can be used (Hoffman et al., 1989).

- *A motor skill–learning approach rather than a cognitive-linguistic approach* to treatment is recommended to emphasize practice at different levels of linguistic complexity (see Chapters 1 and 2). The clinician should avoid isolation practice in favor of contextual practice at syllable, word, phrase, sentence, and conversational levels. The rationale is to provide systematic practice so that numerous opportunities exist to provide the client with internal feedback and clinician-provided knowledge of results.

- The clinician must be cognizant of *coexisting communication problems* and the need for possible therapeutic intervention. Language, literacy skills, and phonological awareness may need to be targeted during the course of the client's treatment.

- Treatment needs to be carried out on a *frequent basis*. Intensive treatment for periods of three to five times per week allow for distributed practice that emphasizes motor planning and production.

- *Home practice* is an important component in treatment if the client's caregivers are willing to conduct home practice sessions. Caregivers willing to participate need training before the introduction of home practice.

- In most cases the *primary aim of therapy is the attainment of intelligibility,* not completely normal speech. The clinician should manipulate the prosodic aspects of speech in training. **Prosody** is the suprasegmental component of speech that is used to signal linguistic and emotional features during speech production. Primary suprasegmental features include the following: (1) syllable stress, (2) intonation, and (3) rate and rhythm. **Naturalness** is a perceptual term used to describe the adequacy or inadequacy of prosody for a particular speaker. The clinician should emphasize word stress and phrase-sentence intonation patterns. Compensatory strategies such as pauses may be instituted with the use of vowel prolongations and the insertion of the *schwa* in speech sound clusters. Speaking rate may also be manipulated so that the client practices at a slower rate. Speaking rate may help improve intelligibility but be perceived as unnatural by normal speakers.

Clinicians should use the systematic use of rhythm, intonation, stress, and accompanying motor movements in speech practice. Some clinicians advocate rhymes and songs as agents in practice. Rhythm drills can be executed through simultaneous speech and body motor movement. For instance, the clinician could have a client practice while maintaining a beat with a drum or some other motor activity.

- The clinician should *emphasize metaphonological analysis and self-monitoring* and attempt to develop these skills with the client. Engaging in the analysis of where a sound is made in the oral cavity and judging the accuracy of productions are important components of treatment. Clinicians need to be mindful of the fact that introspective skills such as these are used with clients who are approximately 5 to 6 years of age and older.

- The clinician should *limit the number of training stimuli* so that a small number of practice items exist for a specific task. The clinician should ensure that drill activities are intensive but distributed (rather than executed in massed practice periods) and formulate multiple production goals so that each can be practiced in an individual practice session. In addition, the clinician should extend practice to other situations and different caregivers who interact with the client.

- It may be useful to furnish *multisensory stimulation* to the client. Rather than simply using an auditory model, other forms of input such as touch or visual cueing may also be paired with speech production. More formal methods such as signing and different types of high- or low-technology augmentative and alternative assistive devices may be used. The type and degree of stimulation will depend on the client.

- *Phonotactic constraints* are the rules of a language that govern permissible word and syllable shapes. The clinician should consider these constraints when developing treatment stimuli (see Chapter 2). For example, Velleman (1994) provides an example of a specific activity that was used with a child diagnosed with CAS. To introduce and practice CV syllable shapes, a "baba board" was devised. Pictures were placed on a board, and CV shapes were used as the initial verbal representations of the stimuli. For example, /bæ:/-sheep, /mʊ:/ -cow, /bʊ:/-ghost, and /ni:/-knee were associations that were used. Using this technique, the clinician points to a picture and the child produces the CV representation. The child also produces repetitions of the same stimuli and is asked to self-monitor the accuracy of productions.

Velleman and Strand (1994) propose that practice in an individual session be divided into the following four different treatment activities:

1. The clinician begins the session with activities that require the client to imitate body or oral motor sequence patterns (or both). This is a readiness activity for the activities that are to follow.

2. Syllable sequence practice activities are then introduced with segmentals and syllable shapes that the child uses. The clinician uses sequences that differ according to articulatory position (/budugu/ or *buy two goats*) to vary practice and facilitate motor planning.

3. Single-word items are introduced to build a core vocabulary of intelligible words.

4. Sentence practice frames are introduced as a production activity. The clinician begins the activity with a standard carrier phrase; then he or she changes individual words while manipulating the length and complexity of the sentences.

Bernhardt (1994) discusses a number of techniques based on nonlinear phonology that may be used to develop syllable, word, and phrase structure. Some examples include the following:

• In some cases, clients show restrictions in the number of phonemes that they use in the creation of syllables. Bernhardt (1994) recommends that the clinician create an awareness of various syllable and word units through listening activities such as poems that emphasize the syllable of interest. For instance, the clinician initially introduces a new syllable shape (CVC) that the client is not using via a poem. The target items are emphasized to create an awareness on the part of the client for the new syllable as opposed to the client's existing shapes. Before presenting the poem, the client has been introduced to polar opposites such as *big and little* or *long and short* for the purpose of creating a contrast between and among syllable shapes (CV versus CVC). The new shape (CVC/long) can be contrasted with the existing shape (CV/short). The listening and awareness is then followed by production tasks. Bernhardt (1994) recommends that the child make the addition of segments to create CVC shapes from existing syllable shapes (mi → mit).

- Some children exhibit onset or rhyme restrictions. In nonlinear phonology the syllable is divided into the onset and rhyme. The *onset* includes all segments before the resonating segment, which is generally the vowel or resonant nucleus of the syllable. The *rhyme* encompasses the resonating segment and all segments that follow. For example, /st/ is the onset and /ip/ is the rhyme in the word /stip/. If the client deleted the final consonant, then treatment would begin by creating an awareness of the onset and rhyme patterns. Bernhardt (1994) recommends imagery terms such as *head* or *engine* for the onset and *body* or *coach* for the rhyme. This would be followed by contrasting different rhymes so that the client is exposed to different pairs such as the contrast between rhymes with only the resonating segment and rhymes with a final consonant segment (V versus VC). Initial production activities may begin with VC rhymes, and the final consonant or consonants may or may not be in the child's inventory. This production task would be followed by the introduction of onsets to the VC syllables (CVV).

- If the child has a *coexisting oral apraxia*, treatment may be introduced to develop nonspeech isolated and sequential oral movements. However, the clinician must be aware that no evidence suggests that speech will improve through treatment of the oral apraxia. They are separate domains and require task-specific treatment.

Integral Stimulation

Strand and Skinder (1999) have developed an approach to treatment that is based on principles of motor learning and uses practice procedures directed to sensorimotor planning. It was originally developed for acquired apraxia (Rosenbek et al., 1973), but was adapted by the authors for younger clients. The major features of the approach are that the client responds to various cues and practice response time delays, and the client's response to the treatment dictates the specific stimulus presentation mode. To implement the program, a prospective client must be able to attend, maintain eye contact, and imitate the treatment stimuli (Box 3-4).

Step 1: Direct Imitation

Goal. The production of target items with correct articulation, normal speaking rate, and prosody after direct imitation

The clinician presents the practice stimuli in a direct-imitative manner with a reduced speaking rate. If the client can imitate the stimulus, then

---

BOX 3-4   *Summary of Integral Stimulation Treatment*

Goal 1

To produce target items with correct articulation, normal speaking rate, and prosody after direct imitation

1. The clinician presents practice stimuli in a direct-imitative manner with a reduced speaking rate.
2. If the client can imitate the stimulus, then direct imitation continues and the client is instructed to vary speaking rate and prosody of the target items.
3. If the client cannot imitate the stimulus, then the clinician asks the client to produce the targets simultaneously with the clinician. This continues until the client can produce the target items with correct articulation, normal speaking rate, and prosody.

Goal 2

To produce target items with correct articulation, normal speaking rate, and prosody after delayed imitation of at least 3 seconds

1. The clinician explains the time delays to the client and may develop a signal to indicate when he or she should provide the delayed imitative response.
2. The clinician should initially introduce a 2-second delay and gradually increase it to 3 seconds.
3. Practice should continue until the client can produce the target item with correct articulation, normal speaking rate, and prosody after the delay.

Data from Strand E, Skinder A: Treatment of developmental apraxia of speech: integral stimulation methods. In Caruso A, Strand E, editors: *Clinical management of motor speech disorders of children*, New York, 1999, Thieme.

direct imitation continues with the clinician varying the speaking rate and prosody of the target items. The clinician provides practice trials and manipulates rate and prosody while maintaining correct production of target stimuli. Direct imitation continues until the client can produce the targets with correct articulation, normal speaking rate, and prosody.

If the client cannot correctly imitate the target items, he or she is instructed to produce the targets in concurrent fashion. That is, the client produces the targets simultaneously with the clinician's model. If the client cannot produce the targets simultaneously with the clinician, then a reduced production rate and tactile placement cues are used to achieve correct production. Simultaneous production continues until the client can produce the targets with correct articulation, normal speaking rate, and prosody. At that time the clinician reintroduces the direct-imitation condition.

Step 2: Time Delays

Goal. The production of target items with correct articulation, normal speaking rate, and prosody after delayed imitation of at least 3 seconds

Time delays between the imitative cuing of the clinician and the client's response are now introduced. The clinician explains what is to be done and may develop a signal such as pointing to the client when he or she should give the delayed imitative response. Initially the authors recommend that a 2-second delay be introduced and gradually increased to 3 seconds. The clinician should continue practice trials until the client can produce the target items with correct articulation, normal speaking rate, and prosody after the introduction of the delay.

If the child experiences problems with step 2, the clinician may shorten the delay period or revert back to direct imitation. After a period of practice, the clinician either increases the delay or reintroduces the delay condition, depending on the branch alternative selected.

Completion Criteria

Strand and Skinder (1999) indicate that the clinician should determine completion criteria for a specific goal through daily minitests of the child's performance, not the day-to-day accuracy performance percentages that are typically collected for clients with sound system disorders (see Chapter 1). For example, the clinician is working with the client on establishment of /sp/ clusters in the prevocalic position. A practice group of six word items is used. The clinician is using integral stimulation for the introduction of practice stimuli and tracking performance, or what is known as *response to training trials*. At the end of each session, the clinician again presents the group of words used. Each item is presented only one time. The presentation of the stimuli will depend on the level of practice. When working at the direct-imitative level, the clinician uses an imitative model; when working at the delay plus model level, he or she uses that type of stimulus presentation. The clinician should use the minitest results to determine goal completion. If the child performs at a level of 80% to 90% accuracy for two to three consecutive sessions, then the clinician can introduce a new higher-level goal or other stimulus items.

Additional Treatment Approaches

In addition to the speech production treatment methods discussed, additional approaches have been used that include tactile-kinesthetic facilitation, rhythmic and melodic facilitation, and gestural cueing (Square, 1999). Only limited anecdotal information exists regarding the efficacy of these approaches; these are treatments that use different nonspeech methods or alter the speech output of the client to facilitate communication. Box 3-5 presents examples of the different approaches according to the three categories. The tactile-kinesthetic treatments aim to improve speech motor control through the clinician's digital manipulation of the client's mandible, lips, and tongue. Researchers hypothesize that placement of the articulators by the clinician and simultaneous production of the target enhances the client's oral-sensory perception for speech production. For instance, motokinesthetic speech training (Young and Stichfield-Hawk, 1955) entails stimulation of the /f/ speech sound through use of the following tactile cues that are paired with the clinician's model of the target. The client's lower jaw is placed in a nearly closed position, and the lower lip is positioned in contact with the upper central incisors. Airflow for /f/ production is cued by pushing gently on the diaphragm.

Square (1999) indicates that rhythmic treatments act to reduce the rate of speech and accentuate the stress pattern of the target utterance.

BOX 3-5 *Examples by Category of Additional Treatment Approaches to Childhood Apraxia of Speech*

Tactile-Kinesthetic Treatments
Motokinesthetic speech training
Speech facilitation
Prompting

Rhythmic and Melodic Facilitation
Melodic apraxia treatment
MIT

Gestural Cueing
Adapted cueing
Jordan's gestures
Cued speech

MIT, Melodic intonation therapy.

Melodic facilitation adds another dimension by introducing rapid alterations in pitch via respiratory and laryngeal coordination. Melodic intonation therapy is probably the best-known and most widely used treatments in this category. Originally developed for use with adult nonfluent clients with aphasia (Albert et al., 1973), it has also been used with clients diagnosed with CAS (Helfrich-Miller, 1984). Speech phrases are introduced to clients, and they are instructed to produce them in song-type fashion. While producing the utterances, the client pairs speech production with hand tapping. The method has been changed for CAS clients to encompass a hierarchy of phrases that vary by length and linguistic complexity. In addition, signed English replaces the hand tapping as a pacing agent.

Rhythmic treatments reduce the rate of speech and accentuate the stress pattern of the target utterance.	*Research* Note

Square, 1999.

Finally, gestural systems are used to regulate speech production and provide cues concerning vocal tract configurations and movement excursion of the articulators. For instance, Jordan's gestures (Jordan, 1988) consist of a group of visual symbolic gestures that are used to show the articulatory production features of different phonemes. The gestures are used to augment other treatments also being used with the CAS client. The gestures signal placement and movement of the vocal tract along with laryngeal activity. Gestures are used for those phonemes that are problematic for the client to produce.

Jordan's gestures, a group of visual symbolic gestures, are used to show the articulatory production features of different phonemes.	*Research* Note

Jordan, 1988.

TREATMENT OF DEVELOPMENTAL DYSARTHRIA

Clinicians need to be cognizant of the fact that developmental dysarthria—in some cases such as that associated with cerebral palsy—is a chronic problem that may require long-term management (Love, 1992; Yorkston, 1996). Moreover, few clients undergo remediation to the extent of achieving total phonetic mastery and producing completely intelligible speech. Frequently, persistent problems involve a single component of speech production such as articulation or a cumulative problem with respiration, phonation, resonation, and/or prosody (Hayden, 1994). Expectations for recovery may differ for the client who acquired dysarthria later in life as the result of closed head injury, anoxia, stroke, or tumor (Hodge and Wellman, 1999). The general approach to treating developmental dysarthria is based on theoretical concepts adopted from motor skill learning. The principles of this treatment regimen are incorporated in the phonetic approach (discussed in Chapters 1 and 2).

The reader should also note that, as discussed with CAS, there is a paucity of treatment research, with current treatment concepts based primarily on expert opinion and limited case study data (Hodge and Wellman, 1999; Love, 1992). Each client will have a different cluster of symptoms that is associated with a particular site of lesion. In summary, injury to different neurophysiologic mechanisms that regulate the production or execution of speech movement may adversely affect the strength and timing of muscle contractions (Hodge and Wellman, 1999). Physiological differences may include muscle weakness, with the end result being paresis or paralysis of a spastic or flaccid type, muscle tone problems, incoordination of voluntary movement, and involuntary movement.

Research Note	Injury to different neurophysiologic mechanisms that regulate the production or execution of speech movements may adversely affect the strength and timing of muscle contractions.

Hodge and Wellman, 1999.

As discussed previously, some young clients with developmental dysarthria exhibit severe problems, and the goal of treatment must be altered from a primary emphasis on speech development to communication development. That is, some clients may not be able to acquire productive speech that is intelligible; consequently, some form of augmentative or alternative communication may be needed—in combination with speech or exclusively—to facilitate communication. The clinician must measure performance very carefully so that decisions regarding a reasonable expectation for speech and overall communication are formulated. Although the expectation for the client may change, this change needs to be based on objective measurement data that have been collected by the clinician.

Systems Approach to Treatment

Because multiple components of speech production may be involved in developmental dysarthria, it is beneficial to identify those systems that require clinical intervention (Netsell and Daniel, 1979). Respiration, phonation, resonation, articulation, and prosody are potential targets, depending on the problems exhibited by the client (Duffy, 2005; Strand, 1995). Muscle activity of these systems work in coordinated action to create the air pressures and flows that are converted into the sounds of speech (Figure 3-3). The respiratory system consists of the abdominal muscles, diaphragm, and muscles of the ribcage. The muscles of respiration generate and regulate the respiratory forces from the lungs needed for speech production. Normal speakers are capable of rapid inspiration

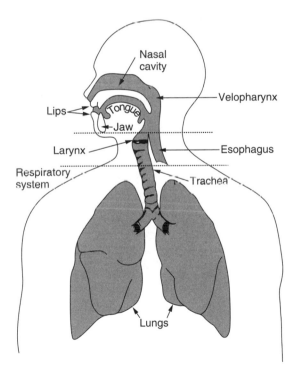

Figure 3-3 ■ Organs of speech production. (Redrawn from Bernthal JE, Bankson NW: *Articulation and phonological disorders,* ed 5, Boston, 2004, Allyn & Bacon.)

and the maintenance of adequate subglottal air pressure to ensure that air is gradually expired during speech production. Hodge and Wellman (1999) indicate that respiratory forces for speech are responsible for the loudness of speech, the number of words produced per breath, the production of word and syllable stress, and the length of pauses between speech breath units. The phonatory system is composed of the larynx and muscles of the larynx. The larynx is a muscular valve that regulates the airstream created by the respiratory system. Its actions create a vibratory source for all sounds that are voiced, the noise sound supply for glottal stops, aspiration of /h/, and whisper. In addition, abduction of the vocal folds allows for the production of voiceless sounds. The muscles of the larynx also change the length and tension of the vocal folds to adjust the pitch, loudness, and quality of the voice.

Research Note	Respiratory forces for speech are responsible for the loudness of speech, the number of words produced per breath, the production of word and syllable stress, and the length of pauses between speech breath units.

Hodge and Wellman, 1999.

The pharyngeal, oral, and nasal cavities are components of the vocal tract that constitute the structures responsible for sound resonation (Strand, 1995). Different muscle activities of these structures selectively modify the sound source through the process of cavity resonance. The pharyngeal and oral cavities form the primary pathway for the transmission of oral sounds, whereas coupling with the nasal cavity furnishes the pathway for the resonation of nasal sounds. The system of articulation involves the placement of sounds primarily through adjustments of the oral articulators (lips, tongue, jaw). Clinicians are generally cognizant of sound placement and can describe the different placements of vowels and consonants. An interaction occurs between resonation and articulation in the production of speech sounds. For example, the production of vowels is governed by the different configurations of the vocal tract that are created by different articulatory configurations of the tongue, lips, or both. The final system component is that of prosody, which signals linguistic and emotional features in speech. Prosodic features or suprasegmentals are production variables that are superimposed on syllables, words, and phrases. Prosody is a composite of pitch, loudness, and timing variations that are used to denote emotional differences, emphasis, and linguistic variation such as word stress. Normal speakers vary pitch, loudness, and timing factors in their production of speech. Respiratory, laryngeal, and articulatory systems interact in the production of prosodic speech features.

Different treatment approaches may be used individually or in combination when using a systems approach to developmental dysarthria (Hodge and Wellman, 1999). For instance, behavioral treatments including various forms of biofeedback may be implemented to target the normalization of neuromotor function. Different drills and speech training techniques are used to improve physiologic function. In addition, compensatory treatments such as different surgical procedures or prosthetic devices may be used to improve function. For instance, a palatal lift may be constructed to improve velopharyngeal closure for speech. Finally, the use of compensatory speaking strategies, such as rate control and overarticulation of speech movements, may also be used to assist the client in achieving a level of intelligibility that is commensurate with his or her potential level of communication.

Postural Stabilization

Initially it may be necessary in some cases to establish appropriate postural positioning before beginning treatment. Hayden and Square (1994) recommend that the first step with some children is the establishment of satisfactory trunk control to facilitate appropriate breath support, enhance sitting skills, and minimize any tone problems of the oral musculature. If positioning of the client is an issue, then assistance from a physical or occupational therapist is necessary before starting speech production treatment. Solomon and Charron (1998) recommend that appropriate positioning consist of an upright sitting posture with the back as straight as possible, the buttocks in contact with the seat of the chair, and achievement of a 90-degree angle of the hip, knee, and foot. Support for the arms may also be necessary for appropriate postural stabilization. In addition, stabilization of the arms may be useful in furnishing a plane for pushing exercises, because pushing with the arms can facilitate the creation of higher air pressure for speech by aiding movement of the chest wall muscles. Pushing with the arms may also help in cases in which laryngeal adduction is a problem.

Research Note

Postural stabilization involves an upright sitting posture with the back as straight as possible, the buttocks in contact with the chair's seat, and a 90-degree angle of the hip, knee, and foot.

Soloman and Charron, 1998.

Respiration

Duffy (2005) summarized the adult literature regarding respiration and concluded that most speakers with dysarthria do not require treatment for respiration. Typical problems seen in speakers with respiratory involvement include a reduction in words per expiratory breath group, lack of variability in the length of a breath group, and inappropriate phrasing. Respiratory treatment may not be necessary if a client (child or adult) can generate at least 5 cm of water pressure for approximately 5 seconds, which is the approximate average of an utterance produced during one expiration.

Hixon and colleagues (1982) developed a simple test to assess this **expiratory function** (Box 3-6). The clinician fills a glass jar or beaker with water and tapes a metric ruler to the outside of the container. The clinician then places a drinking straw in the container, with the straw immersed at the 5-cm depth level. The straw may be attached to the beaker with a paper clip. The client is instructed to blow into the straw while the clinician times the trial. Several trials are conducted to determine whether the client can carry out the task successfully. The testing procedure can also be used therapeutically to aid in developing adequate subglottal air pressure through the use of practice training trials. However, clinicians should remember that this is a nonspeech task and consider the issue of specificity of training (Duffy, 2005). That is, treatment tasks should be related to the desired speech production goal. If nonspeech movements are to be used, then the clinician should ensure that they are closely related to those necessary for speech. In this case

---

BOX 3-6   *Assessing Expiratory Function*

Respiratory treatment may not be necessary if the client can generate at least 5 cm of water pressure for approximately 5 seconds.
1. The clinician fills a glass jar or beaker with water and tapes a metric ruler to the outside of the container.
2. The clinician places a drinking straw in the container, with the straw immersed 5 cm (the straw may be attached to the container with a paper clip).
3. The clinician asks the client to blow into the straw, and the clinician records how long the client can perform the task.

Data from Hixon T, Hawley J, Wilson J: An around-the-house device for the clinical determination of respiratory driving pressure, *J Speech Hear Disord* 47:413, 1982.

the task provides an index to a client's potential for generating adequate subglottal air pressure for speech. Its use as a treatment task may be beneficial, but it has not been examined through empirical testing.

Information regarding respiration problems in children is limited; however, Solomon and Charron (1998) have reviewed the available literature regarding children with cerebral palsy. They indicate that children with spastic cerebral palsy may have diminished strength, limited range of motion, heightened muscle tone, and heightened reflexes. Conversely, children with athetosis may exhibit problems with postural control, timing of organized movement, and regulation of graded movement. Although the characteristics may describe the different subgroups, severity of those characteristics may differ significantly among clients.

Solomon and Charron (1998) suggest that nonspeech muscle-strengthening exercises of the chest wall may enhance the client's capacity to create higher subglottal pressure and a louder voice. Moreover, increased vital capacity and breathing stamina may assist the client in producing additional syllables on one breath and producing speech for increasing time periods, provided that laryngeal, velopharyngeal, and oral articulatory valves are operating appropriately. In their review of the literature, the authors identified several nonspeech techniques for building expiratory muscle strength. For instance, Cerny and colleagues (1997) had subjects wear a facemask that introduced a resistance to expiratory airflow for a period of 6 weeks. The resistance to expiratory airflow created a condition to exercise the respiratory muscles, and performance measures showed improved breath control for speech. Baker and colleagues (2005) also conducted strength training with a group of healthy adults and found that subjects improved their maximum expiratory pressure after completion of the treatment. Implementation of strength building involves the use of simple instrumentation to replicate the training conditions. The same concern of specificity of training that was discussed previously should also be considered for this exercise technique (Sapienza and Wheeler, 2006; Stathopoulos and Duchan, 2006) because this is a nonspeech technique.

Nonspeech muscle-strengthening exercises of the chest wall may enhance the client's capacity to create higher subglottal pressure and a louder voice.

Research Note

Solomon and Charron, 1998.

Solomon and Charron (1998) also describe a technique designed to improve the coordination of breathing that is known as **inspiratory checking.** The client is instructed to inhale deeply and then exhale slowly when producing speech. The rationale for the technique is that the deep inhalation creates higher lung volume with the potential of having greater subglottal air pressure accessible for speech production. If the technique is too difficult for a client, then it can be carried out without speech; speech can be gradually introduced as the client develops improved breath control.

A final respiratory control technique known as *speech phrasing* is designed to assist the client in replenishing respiratory airflow by alternating between short phrases and frequent inhalations of air (Love, 1992). The client is instructed to produce individual words or short phrases between inhalations. The inhalations are more frequent than normal so that clients can replenish their air supply on a more frequent basis. Love cautions that the client must understand the task and be trained to alternate between short phrasing and breath intake. The technique, which also acts to reduce the speaking rate, allows the client with respiratory problems to produce speech without a significant loss of intelligibility. In some cases a pacing board is used to develop appropriate phrasing (Helm, 1979). The pacing board consists of a small board with a series of slots. The board is placed in front of the client, and he or she touches a slot with a finger when producing a word or short phrase. The external pacing with the finger on the board signals the client to sustain the designated rate of speech.

Phonation

Love (1992) discussed the phonatory problems of young clients with dysarthria and indicated that voice disorders have been described in the literature. Although few treatment data exist, expert opinion suggests that voice disorders remain difficult to treat with behavioral therapy. Despite the negative prognosis, Love recommends a trial period of treatment to determine whether voice therapy is beneficial for a particular client.

Hodge and Wellman (1999) indicate that the coordination of expiration with laryngeal voicing is often problematic for clients with developmental dysarthria. Voicing occurs when the client can adduct the vocal folds in the presence of adequate subglottal air pressure. If adduction is a problem, with the voice weak and breathy, then pushing with the hands in resistance exercises such as holding the sides of a chair or pushing on the top of a table may improve vocal fold approximation and facilitate vocal fold vibration. Another technique is to interconnect the hands and pull outward. If adequate vocal fold vibration is established, then activities to extend phonatory and respiratory control may be introduced at a practice level appropriate to the client. In some cases the client may need to use the pushing technique with vowels in isolation and then move to diphthongs, syllables, words, sentences, and connected speech as individual training criteria are met. Clinicians must carefully monitor treatment to ensure that no laryngeal irritation occurs and that the speaker does not develop any unwanted inappropriate compensatory movements. In addition, Solomon and Charron (1998) caution that effortful closure activities be used carefully with clients who have spastic cerebral palsy. If used therapeutically, then the clinician should use pushing techniques in conjunction with relaxation, muscle-lengthening procedures, and facilitation of normal patterns of movement.

In some cases such as cerebral palsy, hyperadduction of the vocal folds occurs and voice quality is harsh, strained, or both (Academy of Neurologic Communication Disorders and Sciences, 2002). Traditional voice relaxation techniques such as the yawn-sigh, chewing, or chanting may be introduced (Boone and McFarlane, 1994). If a relaxation technique reduces vocal fold hyperadduction, then the improved phonatory adduction may be used in a hierarchy beginning with vowels and eventually transferring production to connected speech.

Resonation

Hypernasality is the primary resonance problem that is seen in clients with involvement of the velopharyngeal mechanism (Duffy, 2005). This problem is perception of unwanted nasal resonance during the production of vowels and other oral vocalic segments. Continuous coupling of the vocal tract with the velopharyngeal port makes speaking inefficient and may stress marginal respiratory and laryngeal systems, resulting in the need for more frequent inhalation and reduced phrasing. In addition, overall vocal loudness may be reduced because of the dampening effect of the nasal cavities, and the presence of nasal emission (articulation problem) may adversely affect intelligibility. Behavioral management of velopharyngeal inadequacy through nonspeech techniques such as blowing, sucking, and swallowing has not been successful (Ruscello, 2004; Yorkston et al., 2001). To date, only one treatment targets strength development through speech production (Kuehn, 1991, 1997; Kuehn et al. 2000; Liss et al., 1994). Kuehn and associates use **continuous positive airway pressure (CPAP)** to apply a resistive load to the velum while producing speech stimuli. CPAP instrumentation generates air pressure from an external generator source to the nasal cavities (channeled via a mask). The external pressure and vocal tract pressure generate two pressure heads that are isolated, provided that velopharyngeal closure is achieved. The use of the external pressure source provides a condition in which a resistance to velar movement is established. Thus a client may practice speech production tasks while the velum is subject to resistance. This enables strength building during speech and is consistent with principles of task specificity (Clark, 2003; Duffy, 2005). That is, the designed exercise activities are explicit to the goal of the muscle rehabilitation program (Clark, 2003; Duffy, 2005). Kuehn and colleagues reported improvement in some of the subjects with motor speech disorders who underwent the CPAP treatment (Liss et al., 1994).

Research Note	To date, only one treatment targets strength development of the velopharyngeal mechanism through speech production: CPAP.

Kuehn, 1991, 1997.

For most clients, management of hypernasality (resonation) and nasal emission (articulation) is achieved through either surgery or the fitting of a **prosthesis.** Davison and colleagues (1990), as cited in Hodge and Wellman (1999), reported the results of surgical intervention with 16 children who had velopharyngeal inadequacy because of neurological disorders. Each underwent a **pharyngoplasty** that was based on presurgical endoscopic findings. After surgery, the subjects received treatment to improve oral articulation errors and breath pressure. Ratings of the children's speech after they received this intervention indicated that a majority improved their intelligibility. The authors reported that the more successful surgical clients displayed satisfactory presurgical lip and tongue function; however, sufficient evidence does not exist to recommend surgical intervention as a routine procedure for clients with dysarthria (Yorkston et al., 2001).

The **palatal lift** has a significant history in the treatment of velopharyngeal inadequacy because of neurological involvement of the velum (Duffy, 2005). A dental specialist known as a **prosthodontist** constructs an appliance in consultation with a speech-language pathologist. The appliance consists of a palatal portion that fits the configuration of the palate and generally is attached to the upper teeth with clasps. The lift portion is in contact with the soft palate and lifts or elevates the soft palate so that the structure is in approximate contact with the lateral and posterior pharyngeal walls (Figure 3-4). After the appliance is made, the

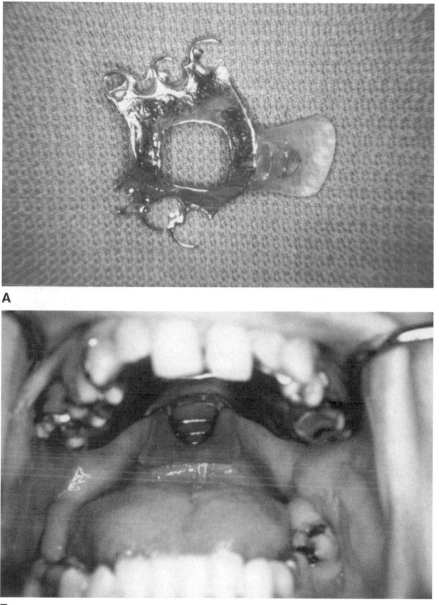

Figure 3-4 ■ Palatal lift prosthesis. **A,** Palatal portion with fasteners and extended lift portion. **B,** Prosthesis in place. (From Duffy JR: *Motor speech disorders: substrates, differential diagnosis, and treatment,* ed 2, St Louis, 2005, Elsevier.)

palatal portion is generally extended over several fitting sessions. Yorkston and colleagues (2001) indicate that clients with flaccid dysarthria are better candidates for a palatal lift than other types of dysarthria. The use of palatal lifts for young clients with developmental dysarthria has not been examined extensively.

Articulation

Treatment of sound system errors is generally a major goal in the intervention of clients with developmental dysarthria. Numerous techniques and procedures have been used to improve production skills, thus influencing intelligibility positively. The discussion of articulation treatment includes (1) direct treatment of sound errors, (2) the use of contrast and intelligibility drills, (3) the use of speech aids, (4) biofeedback treatments, and (5) the manipulation of production variables such as rate of speech and increasing speech effort (Box 3-7). These different treatment techniques are discussed individually, but they are generally used in combination with other systems treatments because the needs of individual clients vary in reference to lesion site and severity of neurological damage.

Duffy (2005) indicates that treatment of developmental dysarthria incorporates different forms of sound system treatment. Because perceived errors are frequently identified as distortions, phonetic placement instructions are used to assist the client in achieving correct production of target sounds. Once a target sound has been developed in isolation or syllables, transfer to other contexts may be carried out; Duffy recommends that integral stimulation—discussed earlier in this chapter (Strand and Skinder, 1999)—be used as the means to elicit targets and furnish appropriate feedback to the client.

A key issue in sound system training is the appropriateness of different muscle-training techniques such as strength building, relaxation, and stretching, in addition to considering whether the clinician works

---

BOX 3-7 *Sound System Treatment Components*

- Direct treatment of sound system errors
- Contrast and intelligibility drills
- Speech aids
- Biofeedback treatments
- Manipulation of production variables, such as rate of speech and increasing speech effort

in a nonspeech or speech mode during treatment. Duffy (2005) indicates that during speech, speakers use approximately 10% to 30% of the maximum muscle force of the lips and tongue and about 2% of the available jaw muscle force. Moreover, available data from motor learning indicate that muscle treatment be carried out in the context of the goal of treatment. That is, if speech production skills are deficient, then the clinician should target speech production tasks. For example, speech drills might include trials wherein the person maintains the articulatory placement for a brief period of time. A bilabial in the prevocalic position *(pie)* could be held for a brief period of time before release. Jaw opening could be exaggerated using a low vowel transition from lip closure *(pam)* to exercise the jaw-opening muscles and return to lip closure. The examples are activities that may build strength and allow muscle stretching in the context of speech tasks. Duffy (2005) writes that the client be instructed to heighten effort and reduce rate, because these techniques may help attempts at exaggeration. Clinicians can devise different tasks such as the examples described. However, they should caution the client against extensive overexaggeration so that unwanted compensations do not occur.

During speech, speakers use approximately 10% to 30% of the maximum muscle forces of the lips and tongue and approximately 2% of the available jaw muscle force.

Research Note

Duffy, 2005.

Contrastive drills may also be used to assist the client in developing distinctions between manner, place, and voicing problems (Yorkston et al., 1999). The rationale for contrastive drills is not to change a specific production feature difference but to have the client modify speech based on internal analysis of the speech problem. Therefore this is a discovery step for clients and requires them to use their metaphonological analysis skills. The clinician furnishes the client with appropriate information so that the appropriate adjustments or compensations may be made. For example, the authors cite a study by DeFeo and Shaefer (1983) wherein a young client with Moebius syndrome received sound system treatment. The client was given a model for bilabial sound productions, whereupon he or she developed a linguadental point of production for /m, p, b, f/. The clinician followed this with contrastive drills between the now linguadental stops and alveolar stops. The client contrasted the pairs by producing /p/ and /b/ with more articulatory force than the alveolars /t/ and /d/. Because lip movement for the bilabials was problematic, the client developed a compensation that did not significantly affect intelligibility. It was a supplementary treatment step that involved contrasting the new target position with an existing target position. The same contrast could also be done with the nasals /m/ and /n/ because /m/ was also produced in a compensatory place of articulation.

Yorkston and colleagues (1999) formulated another treatment activity that they use to improve the client's intelligibility. **Intelligibility drills** consist of word sets that differ by an individual phoneme *(beet, peat, meet, seat, sheet, cheat)*. The words are written individually on cards, and the cards are shuffled. Young clients who have difficulty reading can use pictures. The client then produces the contrastive items individually. The clinician is not aware of the client's selections but is required to identify the words produced. If a correct identification does not occur on the first trial, then the client is given another opportunity to produce the target. If the clinician does not identify the target on the repeat, then the client is instructed to use additional cues such as gesture to assist the clinician in identification. Hodge and Wellman (1999) have modified the drill procedure to include a display board that contains either pictures or graphic representations of the target words. After the client produces the target, the clinician points to the target picture or graphic representation. Yorkston and colleagues (1999) indicate that intelligibility drills are very useful because they prompt the client to experiment and develop ways to produce perceptually acceptable speech. The drills also allow the clinician to adjust the task to meet the level of the client's intelligibility. Finally, the drills place the client in situations that may involve communication breakdowns that he or she must resolve.

Speech aids or prostheses are sometimes used to assist the client in the production of various articulatory placements. Generally the use of a palatal lift (discussed under Resonation) is used when considering the use of a prosthesis; however, other intraoral devices have been developed for dysarthric speakers (Light, 1995). The palatal augmentation prosthesis may be of assistance to clients with degenerative motor disease. The device is worn intraorally and is designed to compensate for decreased range of tongue motion. The prosthesis is shaped to provide contact points for the tongue and minimize the effect of lingual dysfunction on speech and swallowing. The **bite block** is another device that is used with developmental dysarthria clients (Duffy, 2005). The device is constructed of acrylic material and placed in the lateral portion of the mouth so that the bite block is in contact with the upper and lower teeth. The client is instructed to bite the block while speaking in therapy. The rationale is that the bite block acts to stabilize the jaw and enable movement of the lips and tongue without interference. A variation of a bite block may be used in trial fashion to determine whether it might be appropriate for a client. A tongue blade may be inserted between the upper and lower canines. Netsell (1985) suggests that the width of the blade be trimmed to approximately 5 to 8 mm for children. The client is instructed to bite down gently on the blade. With stabilization of the jaw, labial and lingual articulations may be examined in the context of different phonetic environments.

Biofeedback has been used quite extensively in the treatment of sound system errors and other speech and swallowing disorders (Crary and Groher, 2000; McGuire, 1995; Volin, 1998). Performance information that generally is not available on a conscious basis is provided via instrumentation so that the learner may modify his or her current performance. Davis and Drichta (1980) describe biofeedback as the provision of real-time information regarding a specific physiologic system that is under neurologic control but not accurately perceived by the learner. Biofeedback is useful because it makes ambiguous sensory information available to the learner, and the appropriate modifications in performance may be made. (See Chapter 6 for a detailed discussion of biofeedback applications.)

Biofeedback is the provision of real-time information regarding a specific physiologic system that is under neurologic control but not accurately perceived by the learner.

Research Note

Davis and Drichta, 1980.

Manipulation of speaking rate and effort are production variables frequently targeted in therapy for clients with developmental dysarthria (Hodge and Wellman, 1999). The underlying purpose is to improve the client's intelligibility. Speaking rate is a composite of articulatory production and pauses. According to Yorkston and colleagues (1999), articulatory production times are consistent within speakers, but pause times will vary considerably. Speaking rates for normal speakers vary as a function of the specific speaking task. Normal rates average from 160 to 170 words per minute (wpm) for a paragraph-reading task and approximately 190 wpm for individual sentence reading. Data for conversational speech show considerable variance, with recorded speaking rates ranging from 150 to 250 wpm. A reduction in speaking rate may be helpful for some speakers, but general improvement in intelligibility is not found for all speakers (Yorkston et al., 1999). Another factor to be considered in altering rate is speech naturalness. In some cases a slower speaking rate has a significant effect on the way a speaker's speech is perceived as being natural or unnatural.

Although most speakers with dysarthria speak at a slower rate, Yorkston and colleagues (1999) believe that speakers with either hypokinetic or ataxic dysarthria are the best candidates for rate control therapy. The client should receive a period of trial therapy to assess the effect of rate control on intelligibility and speech naturalness. Different pacing techniques such as a pacing board (previously described) and an alphabet board can be used. The alphabet board technique requires the client to identify the first letter of each word spoken on the board. **Delayed auditory feedback (DAF)** is another treatment that has been used to alter rate. Instrumentation is necessary for this to be used with a client. Finally, Yorkston and colleagues (1999) developed rhythmic cueing to reduce rate while minimizing the potential effect of the rate reduction on speech naturalness. Using this technique, the clinician establishes the rate by pointing to words in a written passage in a rhythmic manner. The clinician introduces word rate differences by pointing and taking more time with a word to be emphasized. Pause time is done in the same way; the clinician points to a space to introduce an appropriate pause. This technique helps to maintain speech naturalness but can only be done with printed passages. Rhythmic cueing has been computerized so that word cues and pause times are inserted as part of a selected speaking rate (Beukelman et al., 1997).

Prosody

Duffy (2005) states that the treatment of prosody may improve intelligibility with severe clients and maintain speech naturalness in clients with mild involvement. Prosody is the suprasegmental component of speech that speakers use to signify different linguistic and emotional features. The **suprasegmentals** include (1) syllable stress, (2) intonation, and (3) rate and rhythm (Kehoe and Stoel-Gammon, 1997; Kent, 1998). *Naturalness* is a perceptual term used to describe the adequacy or inadequacy of prosody for a given speaker. Yorkston and colleagues (1999) explain that speech is perceived as natural if the speech is consistent with a listener's internal values of stress, intonation, and rate and rhythm. Physiologically, syllable stress is achieved through the use of increased effort compared with other syllables in an utterance, whereas intonation is regulated by respiratory or laryngeal actions (or both). Rate and rhythm is the marker of speech movement velocities and patterns. Prosodic features are coded through the interaction of the different speech production systems, which have been discussed.

Speech is perceived as natural if consistent with a listener's internal values of stress, intonation, and rate and rhythm.	*Research* Note

Yorkston et al., 1999.

Some clinicians feel that prosody may improve if treatment is directed to an awareness and maximum use of the breath group according to the ability of the client (Duffy, 2005). The breath group functions as a primary component of prosody. In normals, the breath group is more closely related to the syntax of the utterance than the physiologic process of respiration. The speaker with respiratory or laryngeal control problems (or both) may have problems of prosody and need to improve respiratory and phonatory control for speech. (Recommendations for treatment are contained in the sections on Respiration and Phonation.) Clients with respiratory and phonatory problems may need to be taught to "chunk" utterances at appropriate syntactic boundaries within their limited breath groups. That is, if respiration, phonation, or both remain problematic, then clients can be taught the compensatory strategy of chunking utterances at important syntactic boundaries. This aids the listener in comprehending the message, and the client's speech may be perceived as more natural.

Another prosody task described by Duffy (2005) is that of **contrastive stress practice.** Utterances that do not vary in terms of segmental features are used to contrast different prosodic patterns. For instance, the clinician may establish a focal response for the client such as "Jill does not like Karen." The client then uses the focal response to ask a series of questions, such as "does Jill like Karen?" or "does Karen like Fred?" This enables the speaker to use the focal response but vary the prominence of the different syllables. Intonation can also be targeted with a focal response. The client would need to answer with different intonation shifts to signal questions (rising intonation at the end of the utterances) or statements (falling intonation at the end of an utterance).

Referential speaking tasks are also used to assist clients with prosody (Duffy, 2005). For instance, the clinician might prepare a list of phrases or sentences with predetermined stress on certain targets. The material is randomized, and the client reads it to a listener who is not familiar with the material. The listener's role is to identify those targets in the reading material. For instance, phrases such as *a big green house* versus *a big greenhouse* would be randomly organized and read by the client. The task of the listener is to identify the appropriate meaning associated with each phrase. The same can be done with sentences and extended to multiple prosodic targets of phrasing, intonation, and stress. For example, statements such as "the cow herd will move deer" versus "the cow heard Will move dear" versus "the cow herd will move, dear" can be constructed for practice purposes.

SUMMARY

Treating clients with developmental motor speech disorders is a very challenging task for the clinician. CAS is conceptualized in the chapter as a motor-planning problem, whereas developmental dysarthria is discussed as a problem of motor execution. The profession is just beginning to understand these disorders; consequently, treatment is based largely on expert opinion and a limited amount of case study data. This cannot and should not deter the clinician from providing treatment services to these clients. Although this chapter deals primarily with sound system disorders, it emphasizes that clients are at risk for language and literacy problems and that clinicians need to be cognizant of this fact. This chapter also explains that speech development may be limited for some clients, which necessitates the use of an augmentative and/or alternative communication system to augment or be used in place of speech output. Careful measurement of speech production goals and caregiver involvement are important factors in optimizing the client's communication skills.

CAS is a controversial disorder in terms of identification, and it appears that many clients are being diagnosed with CAS at a very young age. Although definitive markers of CAS are not clearly established, some markers or clusters of symptoms help the clinician in diagnosis and treatment of the disorder. If the practitioner is in doubt regarding the diagnosis of CAS, then he or she should engage in diagnostic therapy. In this case the client is not given a diagnosis but is enrolled for a short period of diagnostic treatment to determine whether the diagnosis of CAS is appropriate. The techniques and procedures discussed in this chapter are directed to treatment of the sound system and prosody of speech.

Clients with developmental dysarthria exhibit different speech symptoms that vary as a function of the lesion site and the severity of neurologic involvement. In addition, nonspeech behaviors such as feeding and swallowing are problematic for these individuals. Clients may exhibit mild or severe disorders of respiration, phonation, resonation, articulation, and prosody; therefore it is important to employ a systems approach to diagnosis and treatment. Although this chapter discusses different treatment methods for each system, the systems work in synchrony to produce perceptually acceptable speech. Consequently, the clinician will generally need to incorporate a variety of methods to meet the needs of a specific client.

REFERENCES

Academy of Neurologic Communication Disorders and Sciences: *Practice guidelines for dysarthria: evidence for the behavioral management of the respiratory/phonatory system*, Tech Rep No 3, Minneapolis, 2002, Academy of Neurologic Communication Disorders and Sciences. Available at http://www.ancds.org/practice.html. Accessed July 24, 2006.

Albert M, Sparks R, Helm N: Melodic intonation therapy for aphasia, *Arch Neurol* 29:130-131, 1973.

American Speech-Language-Hearing Association: *Childhood apraxia of speech* [technical report], Rockville, Md, 2006, American Speech-Language-Hearing Association. Available at http://www.asha.org. Accessed February 5, 2007.

Bahr RH, Velleman SI, Ziegler MA: Meeting the challenge of suspected developmental apraxia of speech through inclusion, *Top Lang Disord* 19:19-35, 1999.

Baker S, Davenport P, Sapienza C: Examination of strength training and detraining effects in expiratory muscles, *J Speech Lang Hear Res* 48:1325-1333, 2005.

Bernhardt B: Phonological intervention techniques for syllable and word structure development, *Clin Commun Disord* 4:54-65, 1994.

Beukelman DR, Yorkston K, Tice R: *Pacer/tally rate measurement software*, Lincoln, Neb, 1997, Tice Technology Services.

Boone DR, McFarland S: *The voice and voice therapy*, ed 5, Englewood Cliffs, NJ, 1994, Prentice Hall.

Campbell TF: Functional treatment outcomes in young children with motor speech disorders. In Caruso A, Strand E, editors: *Clinical management of motor speech disorders of children*, New York, 1999, Thieme.

Caruso A, Strand E: Motor speech disorders in children: definitions, background and a theoretical framework. In Caruso A, Strand E, editors: *Clinical management of motor speech disorders of children*, New York, 1999, Thieme.

Cerny FJ, Panzarella KJ, Stathopoulos E: Expiratory muscle conditioning in hypotonic children with low vocal intensity, *J Med Speech Lang Pathol* 5:141-152, 1997.

Clark HM: Neuromuscular treatments for speech and swallowing: a tutorial, *Am J Speech Lang Pathol* 12:400-415, 2003.

Crary MA, Groher ME: Basic concepts of surface electromyographic biofeedback in the treatment of dysphagia: a tutorial, *Am J Speech Lang Pathol* 9:116-125, 2000.

Cumley GD, Swanson S: Augmentative and alternative communication options for children with developmental apraxia of speech: three cases studies, *Augment Altern Commun* 15:110-125, 1999.

Davis SM, Drichta CE: Biofeedback: theory and application to speech pathology. In Lass N, editor: *Speech and language advances in basic research and practice,* New York, 1980, Academic Press.

Davis BL, Jakielski KJ, Marquardt TP: Developmental apraxia of speech: determiners of differential diagnosis, *Clin Linguist Phon* 12:25-45, 1998.

Davis BL, Velleman SL: Differential diagnosis and treatment of developmental apraxia of speech in infants and toddlers, *Infant-Toddler Intervention* 10:177-192, 2000.

Davison P, Razzell R, Watson H: The role of pharyngoplasty in congenital neurogenic speech disorders, *Br J Plastic Surg* 43:187-196, 1990.

DeFeo AB, Schaefer CM: Bilateral facial paralysis in a preschool child: oral-facial and articulatory characteristics: a case study. In Berry W, editor: *Clinical dysarthria,* Austin, Tex, 1983, Pro-Ed.

Duffy JR: *Motor speech disorders: substrates, differential diagnosis, and management,* ed 2, St Louis, 2005, Elsevier.

Forrest K: Are oral-motor exercises useful in the treatment of phonological/articulatory disorders? *Semin Speech Lang* 23:15-26, 2002.

Hall PK: A letter to the parent(s) of a child with developmental apraxia of speech. IV. Treatment of DAS, *Lang Speech Hear Serv Sch* 31:179-181, 2000.

Hall PK, Jordon LS, Robin DA: *Developmental apraxia of speech: theory and clinical practice,* Austin, Tex, 1993, Pro-Ed.

Hayden D: Differential diagnosis of motor speech dysfunction in children, *Clin Commun Disord* 4:119-141, 1994.

Hayden DA, Square PA: Motor speech treatment hierarchy: a systems approach, *Clin Commun Disord* 4:162-174, 1994.

Helfrich-Miller KR: Melodic intonation therapy with developmentally apraxic children. In Perkins WH, Northern JL, editors: *Seminars in speech and language,* New York, 1984, Thieme-Stratton.

Helm NA: Management of palilalia with a pacing board, *J Speech Hear Disord* 44:350-353, 1979.

Hixon T, Hawley J, Wilson J: An around-the-house device for the clinical determination of respiratory driving pressure, *J Speech Hear Disord* 47:413, 1982.

Hodge MM, Hancock HR: Assessment of children with developmental apraxia of speech: a procedure, *Clin Commun Disord* 4:102-118, 1994.

Hodge MM, Wellman L: Management of children with dysarthria. In Caruso A, Strand E, editors: *Clinical management of motor speech disorders of children,* New York, 1999, Thieme.

Hoffman PR, Schuckers GH, Daniloff RG: *Children's phonetic disorders,* Boston, 1989, College-Hill Press.

Jordan LS: *Gestures for cueing phonemes in verbal apraxia: a case study.* Paper presented at the Annual Meeting of the American Speech-Language-Hearing Association, Boston, 1988.

Kehoe M, Stoel-Gammon C: The acquisition of prosodic structure: an investigation of current accounts of children's prosodic development, *Languages* 3:113-144, 1997.

Kent RD: Prosody in the young child. In Yoder DE, Kent RD, editors: *Decision making in speech-language pathology,* Philadelphia, 1988, BC Decker.

Kent RD: Motor control: neurophysiology and functional development. In Caruso A, Strand E, editors: *Clinical management of motor speech disorders of children,* New York, 1999, Thieme.

Kuehn DP: New therapy for treating hypernasal speech using continuous positive airway pressure (CPAP), *Plast Reconstr Surg* 88:959-966, 1991.

Kuehn DP: The development of a new technique for treating hypernasality: CPAP, *Am J Speech Lang Pathol* 6:5-8, 1997.

Kuehn DP, Imrey PB, Tomes L et al: *Efficacy of continuous positive airway pressure (CPAP) in the treatment of hypernasality.* Paper presented at the Annual Convention of the American Cleft Palate–Craniofacial Association, Atlanta, 2000.

Lewis BA, Freebairn LA, Hansen AJ et al: School-age follow-up with childhood apraxia of speech, *Lang Speech Hear Serv Sch* 35:122-140, 2004.

Light J: A review of oral and oropharyngeal prostheses to facilitate speech and swallowing, *Am J Speech Lang Pathol* 4:15-21, 1995.

Liss JM, Kuehn DP, Hinkle KP: Direct training of velopharyngeal musculature, *J Med Speech Lang Pathol* 2:243-245, 1994.

Love RJ: *Childhood motor speech disability,* New York, 1992, Merrill.

Marquardt TP, Sussman HM: Developmental apraxia of speech: theory and practice. In Vogel D, Cannito MP, editors: *Treating disordered speech motor control,* Austin, Tex, 1991, ProEd.

McCauley R: Translating research into clinical action. In Shriberg LD, Campbell TF, editors: *Proceedings of the 2002 Childhood Apraxia of Speech Research Symposium,* Carlsbad, Calif, 2002, The Hendrix Foundation.

McGuire RA: Computer-based instrumentation: issues in clinical applications, *Lang Speech Hear Serv Sch* 26:223-231, 1995.

Netsell R: Construction and use of a bite-block for the evaluation and treatment of speech disorders, *J Speech Hear Disord* 50:100-109, 1985.

Netsell R, Daniel B: Dysarthria in adults: physiologic approach to rehabilitation, *Arch Phys Med Rehabil* 60:502-508, 1979.

Robin DA: Developmental apraxia of speech: just another motor problem, *Am J Speech Lang Pathol* 1:19-22, 1992.

Robin DA: *Assessment and treatment of DAS.* Short course sponsored by Therapy Services LLC and the West Virginia Speech-Language Hearing Association, Morgantown, WV, 1998.

Rosenbek J, Lemme M, Ahern M et al: A treatment for apraxia of speech in adults, *J Speech Hear Disord* 38:462-472, 1973.

Ruscello DM: Considerations for behavioral treatment of velopharyngeal closure for speech. In Bzoch K, editor: *Communicative disorders related to cleft lip and palate,* ed 5, Austin, Tex, 2004, Pro-Ed.

Sapienza C, Wheeler K: Respiratory muscle strength training: functional outcomes versus plasticity, *Semin Speech Lang* 27:236–244, 2006.

Shriberg LD, Aram DM, Kwiatkowski J: Developmental apraxia of speech. I. Descriptive and theoretical perspectives, *J Speech Hear Res* 40:273-285, 1997.

Solomon NP, Charron S: Speech breathing in able-bodied children and children with cerebral palsy: a review of the literature and implications for clinical intervention, *Am J Speech Lang Pathol* 7:61-78, 1998.

Square PA: Treatment approaches for developmental apraxia of speech, *Clin Commun Disord* 4:151-161, 1994.

Square PA: Treatment of developmental apraxia of speech: tactile-kinesthetic, rhythmic, and gestural approaches. In Caruso A, Strand E, editors: *Clinical management of motor speech disorders of children,* New York, 1999, Thieme.

Stathopoulos E, Duchan JF: History and principles of exercise-based therapy: how they inform our current treatment, *Semin Speech Lang* 27:227–235, 2006.

Strand E: Treatment of motor speech disorders in children, *Semin Speech Lang* 16:126-139, 1995.

Strand E, Debertine P: The efficacy of integral stimulation intervention with developmental apraxia of speech, *J Med Speech Lang Pathol* 8:295-300, 2000.

Strand E, Skinder A: Treatment of developmental apraxia of speech: integral stimulation methods. In Caruso A, Strand E, editors: *Clinical management of motor speech disorders of children,* New York, 1999, Thieme.

Velleman SL: The interaction of phonetics and phonology in developmental verbal dyspraxia: two case studies, *Clin Commun Disord* 4:66-77, 1994.

Velleman SL: *Making phonology functional,* Boston, 1998, Butterworth-Heinemann.

Velleman SL: *Childhood apraxia of speech: resource guide,* Clifton, NY, 2003, Thomson Delmar Learning.

Velleman SL, Strand C: Developmental verbal dysapraxia. In Bernthal JE, Bankson NW, editors: *Child phonology: characteristics, assessment, and intervention with special populations,* New York, 1994, Thieme.

Volin RA: A relationship between stimulability and the efficacy of visual feedback in the training of a respiratory control task, *Am J Speech Lang Pathol* 7:81-90, 1998.

Yorkston KM: Treatment efficacy: dysarthria, *J Speech Hear Res* 39:S46-S57, 1996.

Yorkston KM, Beukelman D, Strand EA et al: *Management of motor speech disorders in children and adults,* ed 2, Austin, Tex, 1999, Pro-Ed.

Yorkston KM, Spencer K, Duffy J et al: Evidence-based practice guidelines for dysarthria: management of velopharyngeal function, *J Med Speech Lang Pathol* 9:257-274, 2001.

Young E, Stichfield-Hawk S: *Motokinesthetic speech training therapy,* Stanford, Calif, 1955, Stanford University Press.

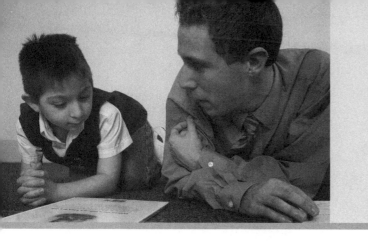

4

Treatment of Children with Structural-Based Disorders

velar fricative
velopharyngeal dysfunction
water manometer
X-linked cleft palate

LEARNING GOALS ▰▰▰▰

■ Define and provide examples of the following four types of errors in speech sound production: (1) developmental errors, (2) obligatory errors, (3) compensatory errors, and (4) phoneme-specific nasal emission.

■ Describe the general treatment concepts for children with cleft lip and palate.

■ Describe a general treatment plan for children with compensatory errors.

■ Discuss several types of performance feedback used in the treatment of sound system errors, and outline the progression of steps involved in this treatment.

■ Discuss other oral structural deficits in addition to cleft lip and palate, and discuss several treatment considerations related to each.

Some clients with articulation and phonological disorders have anomalies of the oral speech mechanism. These can be minor variations, such as missing teeth, or major problems, such as cleft palate. Treatment needs to be individualized for these children, and specific intervention protocols are presented in this chapter in relation to different structural problems.

Before reviewing treatment concepts for children with structural-based disorders, the reader must understand that treatment will differ according to the sound system errors identified in the child's speech. The structural problem may be minor in nature, such as missing incisor teeth, or it may be major, such as cleft lip and palate. Although the major aim of this chapter is to address children with **cleft lip and palate** (Figure 4-1), treatment recommendations are also provided for other structural variations that the practitioner may see infrequently. Clinicians need to be cognizant of the fact that variations in anatomy (structure or structures) can influence the physiology (function or functions) of speech sound production (Ruscello, 2001; St. Louis and Ruscello, 2000). Consequently, analysis of a client's speech sound productions needs to be undertaken and the sound production errors classified according to the type of error. Golding-Kushner (2001, 2004) has provided a very useful framework for identifying errors through analysis according to the traditional features of voicing, place, and manner of articulation. After the errors have been identified, they need to be classified as *developmental, obligatory,* or *compensatory.* Table 4-1 summarizes the different error types.

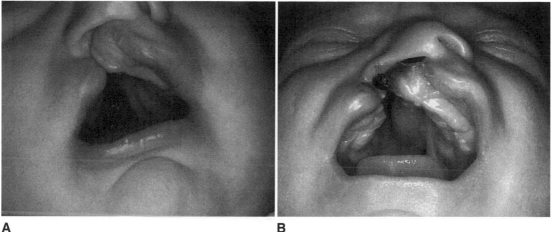

A   **B**

Figure 4-1 ■ Two infants with complete right unilateral cleft lip and palate. **A,** The cleft is complete,
although the cleft segment of the lip and alveolus
is abutting the noncleft segment. **B,** The vomer
bone is attached to the noncleft segment of the secondary plate on the baby's left side, but no attach-
ment exists on the right side. The reader should
note that the right alar wing (side and root of the
nostril) is severely flattened on both sides. (From
Peterson-Falzone SJ, Hardin-Jones MA, Karnell
MP: *Cleft palate speech,* ed 3, St Louis, 2001,
Mosby.)

Clinicians should keep in mind that variations in anatomy (structure) can influence the physiology (function) of speech sound production.	*Research Note*

Ruscello, 2001; St. Louis and Ruscello, 2000.

SOUND SYSTEM ERRORS

Developmental Errors

Developmental errors constitute normal variations that are found in
children who are acquiring the sound system of English (Bernthal and
Bankson, 2004); the developmental errors are not a function of variations
in the anatomy of the vocal tract. The child may outgrow these sound

Table 4-1
Sound System Errors Often Exhibited by Children with Structural-Based Disorders

ERROR TYPES	DESCRIPTION
Developmental errors	Errors found in speech that *are not related* to structural defects Child may outgrow errors or require treatment (if errors not outgrown)
Obligatory errors	Errors present in speech that *are related* to a variation in oral structure Obligatory errors not amenable to speech treatment When oral structure modified via surgical, orthodontic, or dental treatment, errors generally resolve spontaneously
Compensatory errors	Errors used in substitution of individual sounds or sound classes Speech treatment used to modify production errors

Data from Golding-Kushner KJ: *Therapy techniques for cleft palate speech and related disorders,* San Diego, 2001, Singular.

errors or continue past the developmental period and require treatment if the errors become residual (Ruscello, 2003). For example, a child may exhibit a lingual protrusion, or what is otherwise labeled as a *frontal lisp* of /s, z/. This error is developmental and is not related to a structural deviation of the vocal tract. If it persists past the expected period of developmental variation, then the error becomes a target for treatment. Many sound system errors are developmental and subject to treatment in early elementary school because the child does not spontaneously correct them during the period of expected phonological maturation.

Obligatory Errors

In contrast to developmental errors, **obligatory errors** are the result of a structural problem that influences the physiologic movement or

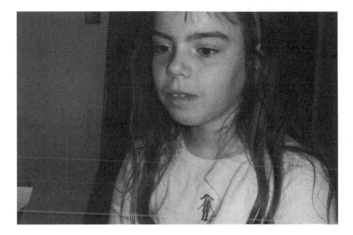

Figure 4-2 ▪ Client shows protrusion of the upper central incisors during lip closure. The teeth are misaligned in a labioverted orientation. Lingual protrusion on the production of alveolar sounds would be classified as *obligatory.*

movements required to correct sound production (Golding-Kushner, 2001; Ruscello et al., 1985; Figure 4-2). Generally the productions are identified perceptually as sound distortions. Some authors such as Kummer (2001a) refer to obligatory errors as **passive speech characteristics.** These errors also may be found in children wearing dental or orthodontic appliances because the devices interfere with the place of articulation. Because obligatory errors are the consequence of an anatomical difference, they will typically not improve with behavioral sound system treatment. However, obligatory errors generally resolve spontaneously when the structural defect has been corrected (Kummer et al., 1989; Moller, 1994). For example, a child with a Class III occlusion shows advancement of the lower jaw or mandible beyond the upper jaw or maxilla. Correct placement of bilabial, labiodental, and alveolar sounds may be problematic because the anatomical defect causes obligatory tongue protrusion. In this case the practitioner would not treat the sound errors but rather refer the child to a dental specialist such as an oral surgeon or orthodontist. After correction via surgery or orthodontic treatment, the production problem should be resolved. That is, a change in oral form typically results in a positive change in oral function (Ruscello et al., 1986; Vallino, 1990).

Research Note	Obligatory errors generally resolve spontaneously once the structural defect involved has been corrected.

Kummer et al., 1989; Moller, 1994.

Children wearing various oral appliances may also demonstrate obligatory errors that occur because of the effects of the oral appliance placement. Production errors resolve when the children become accustomed to the appliance (Marino et al., 2005) or after the appliance has corrected the anatomical defect and has been removed. Obligatory errors may also result from other structural deviations that include missing or crooked teeth, variations in anatomy, and defects of hard and soft palate (Peterson-Falzone, 1988; Peterson-Falzone et al., 2001; Ruscello et al., 2005; Van Borsel et al., 2000).

Children with clefts of the lip and palate exhibit sound production errors, and some of those errors may be obligatory. Kuehn and Moller (2000) indicate that obligatory errors are part of the complex of problems seen in the cleft palate population. Velopharyngeal dysfunction and coexisting variations in oral anatomy cause these errors. In English, all speech sounds (with the exception of the nasals) are produced with velopharyngeal closure. Dynamic movement of the velum and pharyngeal walls acts to separate the nasal cavity from the oral cavity. If velopharyngeal dysfunction occurs because of an anatomic deficiency, then obligatory errors may be present in the child's speech.* Golding-Kushner (2001) lists hypernasality, nasal emission, nasal turbulence, reduced intraoral pressure, and sound distortions caused by the presence of oronasal fistulae as obligatory errors. The reader should note that hypernasality is a resonance disorder (a sequela of velopharyngeal dysfunction, not a sound system error). The disorder involves the perception of unwanted nasal resonance during the production of oral voiced sounds such as vowels and semivowels.

Research Note	Hypernasality, nasal emission, nasal turbulence, reduced intraoral pressure, and sound distortions caused by the presence of oronasal fistulae are examples of obligatory errors in the cleft palate population.

Golding-Kushner, 2001.

*Velopharyngeal dysfunction also may result from neuromuscular impairment, which is discussed in greater detail in Chapter 3.

Nasal emission is the passage of air into the nasal cavity during the production of pressure consonants, plosives, fricatives, and affricates (Peterson-Falzone et al., 2001). Nasal emission may be perceptually audible to the examiner or inaudible. It presents as bursts of air or a continuous stream of air emitted nasally during pressure sound production. Another form of nasal emission is **nasal turbulence.** Air passes through the nasal cavity and may set tissue into vibration, or air is forced into a narrowed constriction (possibly because of a nasal obstruction). This passage of air is perceived as a nasal rustle or turbulent noise. In some cases the child with velopharyngeal dysfunction produces pressure sounds with correct oral placements; however, these sounds may be produced with reduced intraoral pressure. The child attempts to impound air orally, but the velopharyngeal dysfunction prevents the development of adequate intraoral pressure. **Reduced intraoral pressure** may also be present in the speech of children with oronasal fistulae. **Oronasal fistulae** are breakdowns in tissue at the site of surgical closure of the palate (Kummer, 2001a) that result in an opening into the nasal passage. Some small fistulae are asymptomatic, but large fistulae can adversely affect pressure sound production. Occlusion of the nostrils generally results in adequate intraoral pressure buildup for producing pressure sounds in the case of reduced intraoral pressure. To eliminate the obligatory errors, surgical and/or dental intervention is generally necessary.

CASE STUDY 4-1

Obligatory Errors: Phonetic Stimulability Treatment

E.W. is a 3-year, 3-month-old boy who was born with a complete unilateral cleft of the primary and secondary palates. As reported by his mother, he underwent lip repair surgery at the age of 3 months and palate repair surgery at 2 years. The palate repair was delayed because of problems with medical reimbursement. The client received treatment from a plastic surgeon who was not affiliated with an interdisciplinary cleft palate team. At the time of speech assessment, E.W. was noted to have an anterior fistula at the junction of the hard palate and alveolus.

An analysis of the client's speech production indicated a consonant inventory of the plosives /p, b, t, d/, nasals /m, n, ŋ/, liquids /l/, and glides /j, w/, as well as all vowels and diphthongs. E.W. also used all simple syllable shapes. Fricatives and affricates were replaced by /h/, /k, g/ replaced by /n/, and /w/ used in place of /r/. The client was not stimulable for sounds that were not in his inventory. It was noted that the client did not use compensatory articulations such as glottal stops, pharyngeal fricatives, or nasal snorts and had received no speech assessment or treatment before arriving at the clinic for treatment. Hypernasality was identified during the production of vocalic sounds. Audible nasal emission was perceived during the production of the plosives that were used productively. The client did not have a history of middle-ear involvement and passed a pure-tone hearing screening. Clinicians made a management decision to provide a trial period of treatment to assist the client in achieving correct placement of oral speech sounds, with the secondary objective of reevaluating velopharyngeal closure for speech and identifying any possible contributions of the fistula.

Provision of treatment was compounded by the fact that E.W. and his family lived some distance from the clinic, which prevented intensive treatment. As a result, he was scheduled for a 50-minute session once a week for a period of 12 weeks. The stimulability program developed by Miccio (2005) and discussed in Chapter 2 was used for the purpose of expanding the client's phonetic inventory. It also provided a therapeutic milieu that garnered the client's attention and active participation because he was so young. The major goal was developing the fricative and affricate sound classes because they were absent from the child's inventory. As an addition to the treatment, the clinician and child would occlude their nostrils with their fingers when producing target items. This technique enabled the client to impound intraoral air pressure requisite to the production of pressure sounds. The clinician deemed this necessary because of the nasal emission noted during the assessment.

Briefly, the stimulability program targets nonstimulable and stimulable sounds in the contexts of isolation or syllables. Each sound is paired with an animal or object character, as well as a specific body motion or hand gesture. Both stimulable and nonstimulable sounds are introduced to ensure client success. As mentioned previously, the program was very appealing to E.W., and he was very motivated to participate. His mother was taught to carry out the stimulability program and did so each day for approximately 20 minutes. Generalization testing indicated the addition of /f, v, s, k/ in CV words and stimulability in isolation for /z, ʃ/. The stimulability program also provided a focus for the child and a foundation for continued treatment of sound system errors and for monitoring the influence of the fistula and velopharyngeal mechanism on speech.

Commentary

The client continues to exhibit hypernasality, a resonance disorder and nasal emission, an articulatory disorder, and a reduced phonetic inventory, but he did not develop unwanted compensatory errors. This result is unusual because most young clients with hypernasality and nasal emission develop unwanted compensatory errors. The reader should note that these perceptual features are generally indicative of a velopharyngeal closure deficit. Nasal emission is an obligatory error; however, the clinic did provide treatment for it. Until velopharyngeal closure for speech and any contributions of the fistula can be determined through instrumental assessment, the clinician must continue to develop the child's phonetic inventory and minimize the possibility of the client developing unwanted compensatory errors. This is why the stimulability treatment program was introduced and digital nasal occlusion was used when producing the pressure sounds. Future treatment includes instrumental assessment and continued treatment using a motor skill–learning approach. The fistula will need to be repaired. A secondary surgical procedure to improve closure for speech might be needed; however, in the interim the client is developing the appropriate placements for oral consonants with the aid of nasal occlusion. Language skills also need to be monitored during development for children born with cleft palate (and intervention initiated, if necessary). Finally, clients such as E.W. require long-term care from a cleft palate and craniofacial team, which is a recommendation that was also presented to the parents and was implemented with their permission.

Compensatory Errors

Golding Kushner (2001) explains that **compensatory errors** are used in substitution of intended speech sounds or speech sound classes and are sometimes referred to as *active speech characteristics* (Kummer, 2001a). In the case of cleft lip and palate, the causal factors for compensatory errors are **velopharyngeal dysfunction** or oronasal fistulae (Peterson-Falzone et al., 2001). The child attempts to impound air pressure posterior to the point of oral-nasal coupling. Compensatory errors are glottal stops, nasal snorts, velar fricatives, pharyngeal fricatives, pharyngeal stops, and middorsum palatal stops (Figure 4-3). A **glottal stop** is articulated by completely occluding the vocal tract at the level of the vocal folds and then releasing the impounded air pressure. Trost-Cardamone (1990a) points out that a glottal stop may be used in place of oral stops and also substituted for other pressure consonants, including the lingual fricatives and the affricate speech sounds. A **nasal snort** articulation is produced by channeling air directly through the nasal tract. The production is used frequently in place of fricatives. Practitioners can

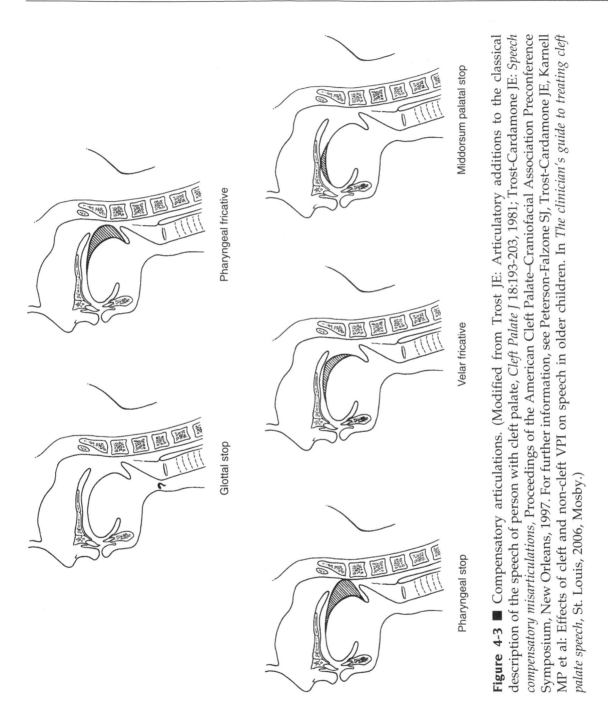

Pharyngeal fricative

Glottal stop

Velar fricative

Middorsum palatal stop

Pharyngeal stop

Figure 4-3 ■ Compensatory articulations. (Modified from Trost JE: Articulatory additions to the classical description of the speech of person with cleft palate, *Cleft Palate J* 18:193-203, 1981; Trost-Cardamone JE: *Speech compensatory misarticulations*, Proceedings of the American Cleft Palate–Craniofacial Association Preconference Symposium, New Orleans, 1997. For further information, see Peterson-Falzone SJ, Trost-Cardamone JE, Karnell MP et al: Effects of cleft and non-cleft VPI on speech in older children. In *The clinician's guide to treating cleft palate speech*, St. Louis, 2006, Mosby.)

differentiate nasal emission from nasal snorting by occluding the child's nostrils during speech production. If the problem is nasal emission, then the sound will be produced in a perceptually acceptable manner. In the case of a nasal snort, no oral articulated sound is made because the nasal snort serves as the substitution for the intended speech sound.

A glottal stop may be used in place of oral stops and also substituted for other pressure consonants, including the lingual fricatives and the affricate speech sounds.	*Research* Note

Trost-Cardamone, 1990a.

Golding-Kushner (1995) explains that creating a constriction of the velum with the tongue dorsum produces a **velar fricative.** Air (or air superimposed with the laryngeal tone in the case of voiced sounds) is channeled through the constriction. Pharyngeal fricatives and stops are produced with a constriction of the posterior area of the tongue and pharyngeal wall. Fricative sounds are produced by channeling air (or air and acoustic energy) through a narrow constriction within the vocal tract, whereas the stops are produced with a complete occlusion and quick release. Velopharyngeal dysfunction or a palatal fistula cause pharyngeal fricatives and stops to be used by some clients. A **pharyngeal fricative** may be used in substitution of lingual fricatives and affricates, whereas a **pharyngeal stop** generally replaces the velar stops /k, g/ (Trost-Cardamone, 1990a).

The final category of maladaptive compensations is the **middorsum palatal stop.** A complete occlusion of the vocal tract is created by tongue blade and palate contact. The point of occlusion is anterior to the velar stops /k, g/ and posterior to the alveolar stops /t, d/. This type of compensatory error may occur in cases of velopharyngeal dysfunction but is present more frequently in cases of oronasal fistulae. The compensatory production pattern results in sound system errors that obscure the perception of the phonemic boundaries between /t/ and /k/ and /d/ and /g/ (Gibbon and Crampin, 2001; Trost, 1981).

In a recent investigation, Hardin-Jones and Jones (2005) examined the resonance and speech production skills of 212 preschool children born with cleft palate. The subjects ranged in age from 2 years, 10 months to 5 years, 6 months. The mean age of the group was 3 years, 6 months (124 boys and 88 girls). Each child was given a standard word test and engaged in a conversational interchange. A total of 37%, or approximately 78 subjects, were rated as having moderate to severe hypernasality or had undergone a secondary surgical procedure to reduce nasality. Fifty-three subjects, or 25% of the group, had compensatory errors. The most frequent compensatory errors identified were glottal stops (25%), glottal fricative /h/ (13%), nasal substitutions (13%), middorsum palatal stops (7%), pharyngeal fricatives (3%), and posterior nasal fricatives (3%). The authors indicate that the resonance and speech outcomes are similar to those found in other recent investigations of preschool- and school-aged subjects. The data illustrate the need for speech intervention in a significant portion of children who have a repaired cleft palate and also indicate the frequency of occurrence of the different compensatory errors.

Research Note	In a study of 212 preschool children born with cleft palate, approximately 25% of the children were identified as using compensatory speech errors. The type and frequency were glottal stops (25%), glottal fricative /h/ (13%), nasal substitutions (13%), middorsum palatal stops (7%), pharyngeal fricatives (3%), and posterior nasal fricatives (3%).

Hardin-Jones and Jones, 2005.

Phoneme-Specific Nasal Emission

One final sound system error is **phoneme-specific nasal emission** (Peterson-Falzone et al., 2001). This problem is not related to a structural defect, rather it is a case of mislearning. The child has a competent velopharyngeal mechanism but articulates a speech sound or class of sounds as a nasal fricative. The problem is often associated with the /s/ speech sound or other lingual fricatives and affricatives. Other pressure sounds are produced correctly, and resonance balance is normal. Phoneme-specific nasal emission is readily amenable to speech treatment because no structural impairment exists.

TREATMENT

It is necessary to first discuss general treatment concepts for children with cleft lip and palate, followed by specific treatment concepts for compensatory speech sound errors such as glottal stops. Golding-Kushner (2001) and Peterson-Falzone and colleagues (2006) provide excellent discussions of sound system disorders that may be present in the speech of children with velopharyngeal insufficiency (VPI). Although some propose that the sound system errors of children with VPI are phonologically based (Chapman, 1993; Pamplona and Ysunza, 1999), the reader should note that a physiologic cause underlies many of the errors. For example, Golding-Kushner (2001) indicates that a glottal stop is a physiologically based error, not a phonologically based error. An alteration in the motor output occurs, rather than an error at the linguistic output level. Trost-Cardamone and Bernthal (1993) wrote the following:

> Although we do not know the extent to which early oral structural deviations associated with cleft palate interfere with acquisition of underlying phonological representations, the child with compensatory substitutions has problems with place features at the surface level. For this reason, the clinician should focus instruction on teaching place contrasts within the vocal tract, for the stops, fricatives, and affricates.

General Treatment Concepts

Box 4-1 summarizes the following treatment concepts:

1. Children with cleft lip and palate are monitored by a cleft palate craniofacial team for tertiary care and receive primary and secondary care within their community. Consequently, collaboration is important in providing quality treatment. Grames (2004) points out that in the case of speech-language pathology services, a child has been monitored from birth and the team's speech-language pathologist makes recommendations for speech and language treatment. In many instances, there can be obstacles to effective collaboration because the practitioner who carries out the treatment does not have extensive experience with such clients, and the care philosophies underlying the two teams differ. The most important factor in collaboration is keeping an open line of communication. In addition, situations may exist in which the two groups may need to collaborate in developing and implementing an effective treatment model (Ruscello et al., 1995). If any doubt exists regarding treatment recommendations, then the practitioner responsible for providing services should consult with the team speech-language pathologist. It may also be beneficial to accompany the child on a visit with the cleft palate team.

2. If the child has successful palatal surgery before the age of 18 months, then speech will generally develop normally. Morris (1992) has indicated that approximately 75% of children undergoing palatal repair develop normal speech.

3. In many cases, children who display velopharyngeal dysfunction after initial palatal surgery will need to undergo a secondary surgical repair, such as a pharyngeal flap or sphincter pharyngoplasty, or be fitted with a speech appliance (Kummer, 2001b). If compensatory articulations are present, then therapy *should not be delayed* until surgery or prosthetic intervention takes place. The type of therapy will vary with the child's chronological age and level of development. The reader should note that some studies have shown the elimination of compensatory errors to have a positive influence on velopharyngeal movement (Henningsson and Isberg, 1986). That is, establishing correct oral placements can facilitate velopharyngeal movement toward closure during speech, but hypernasality and nasal emission may remain to some degree. Hypernasality is a resonance disorder, and nasal emission is an articulatory disorder; both are obligatory because of VPI.

4. Children receiving speech treatment and undergoing secondary surgical repair may resume speech treatment after the doctor's clearance. The clinician does not have to postpone treatment for an extended period after surgery (Golding-Kushner, 2001).

5. Most children with cleft palate do not have a muscle weakness, but may have obligatory and compensatory errors or both. Oral motor treatment techniques such as blowing, sucking, or specific resistance exercises to improve lip or tongue strength are not indicated. Moreover, studies designed to improve velopharyngeal function through oral motor treatment have been largely unsuccessful (Tomes et al., 2004). Current research shows that a very small subset of patients with velopharyngeal dysfunction may benefit from strength training directed to the muscles of the soft palate (Tomes et al., 2004). However, the strength training is conducted during speech production activities, not during nonspeech oral motor activities (Ruscello, 2004).

6. Children with cleft palate are susceptible to middle-ear infections and fluctuating hearing loss (McWilliams et al., 1984). The speech-language pathologist must be cognizant of this potential problem and work with the child's parents, teachers, and other caregivers so that the child receives appropriate medical and audiological services.

7. Children with cleft palate are at an increased risk for language delay (Peterson-Falzone et al., 2001). Initial evaluation and periodic monitoring should occur during the preschool years. Treatment should be initiated if deemed necessary.

> **BOX 4-1** *General Treatment Concepts for Children with Cleft Lip and Palate*
>
> - Collaboration is important in providing quality treatment.
> - Children who have had successful palatal surgery before the age of 18 months generally develop normal speech.
> - Often children who display velopharyngeal dysfunction after initial palatal surgery will need a secondary surgical repair or speech appliance.
> - Children receiving speech treatment and undergoing secondary surgical repair may resume treatment after a doctor's clearance. Postponing treatment for a long period after surgery is not necessary in most cases.
> - Most children with cleft palate do not experience muscle weakness but may have obligatory or compensatory errors (or both). Nonspeech oral motor techniques are not effective in treatment.
> - Children with cleft palate are susceptible to middle-ear infections and fluctuating hearing loss.
> - Children with cleft palate are at an increased risk for language delay.

Approximately 75% of children undergoing palatal repair before the age of 18 months develop normal speech.

Research Note

Morris, 1992.

Treatment of Compensatory Errors

Treatment of compensatory errors uses motor skill–learning principles and the treatment framework discussed in Chapters 1 and 2. Treatment goals are formulated from the results of an assessment that includes measures of word articulation and spontaneous speech. Sound system errors identified through testing are then categorized as *developmental, obligatory,* or *compensatory.* Developmental errors may or may not be potential treatment targets, depending on the age of the client. Obligatory errors are usually not targets because the errors are a function of a structural problem. Referral to appropriate medical or dental specialists is needed for correction of structural problems. After the dental and/or medical treatment, a speech-language evaluation is necessary; however, correct function is often attained with a change in structure (Moller,

1994; Ruscello et al., 1985). Conversely, compensatory errors are identified and targeted for treatment. As discussed previously, compensatory errors include glottal stops, nasal snorts, velar fricatives, pharyngeal fricatives, pharyngeal stops, and middorsum palatal stops. Because the goal is correct production of speech sounds (currently being replaced by more posterior articulations), intensive practice in treatment and at home is paramount to the success of treatment.

Golding-Kushner (2001) suggests a progression in the introduction of consonant phonemes that begins with the introduction of /h/ and is then followed by phonemes in an anterior-to-posterior point of articulation. The suggested order of teaching can be modified in cases when sounds are stimulable, the child is producing some oral sounds that are not potential targets, or the child acquires a sound or sound group that is not in the suggested teaching order. For example, Golding-Kushner recommends that bilabials be introduced before alveolars; however, if alveolar sounds are stimulable, then the clinician may want to target them initially. The recommended order of sound groupings is presented in Table 4-2. There are different sound-teaching techniques for use by the practitioner, and these techniques have been developed in response to the posterior articulations that children with cleft lip and palate use in place of correct oral placements. The reader should note that a substantial amount of empirical data does not support such instructional techniques, rather they are based on the experience of practitioners who have worked extensively with this population.

Treatment of Sound System Errors

Performance Feedback

The clinician needs to be cognizant of the fact that many clients with cleft palate may experience problems in achieving correct placement of target sounds. The compensatory errors may be ingrained and not responsive to imitative models alone. Consequently, it may be necessary to provide clients with additional types of performance feedback or assistance during treatment (Box 4-2). Trost-Cardamone (1990a) suggests that a mirror be used to observe articulatory placements and that diagrams of the articulators be used for illustration purposes. This technique is often effective because the client's auditory monitoring of production trials may be problematic, particularly during the initial stages of sound acquisition. Another technique that may be used is occluding the nostrils. The purpose is to allow the generation of intraoral air pressure and to prevent nasal emission in the production of oral pressure sounds. It also furnishes feedback of unwanted air, acoustic energy, or both passing into the nose (Figure 4-4). The **cul-de-sac**

Table 4-2
Suggested Progression of Consonant Phonemes According to Place of Articulation

PLACE OF ARTICULATION	PHONEMES
Group 1	
Laryngeal	/h/
Group 2	
Bilabial	/m, p, b/
Labiodental	/f, v/
Group 3	
Alveolar	/t, d, n/
Linguadental	/θ, ð/
Alveolar	/s, z/
Group 4	
Velar	/k, g, ŋ/
Group 5	
Palatal	/ʃ, ʒ/
Palatal	/tʃ, dʒ/

Data from Golding-Kushner KJ: *Therapy techniques for cleft palate speech and related disorders*, San Diego, 2001, Singular.

technique can be carried out, with the clinician or the child occluding the nostrils. If the child occludes his or her nostrils, then an additional source of feedback exists in the form of tactile information (Kummer, 2001b). When drill activities are being performed, a nasal clip may be used rather than digital manipulation. Another feedback technique is a "listening tube" to detect the nasal emission of air. The listening tube is a piece of clear plastic tubing; one end is placed in a nostril and the other end is placed near the ear. The child can then perceive unwanted nasal air escape if the air is present.

BOX 4-2   *Types of Performance Feedback during Treatment*

- Mirror to observe articulatory placement
- Diagrams of the articulators
- Occlusion of the nostrils (cul-de-sac technique)
- Nasal clip
- Listening tube
- See Scape
- Water manometer
- Drinking straws
- Air paddle
- Instrumental acoustic and physiologic indices of performance

---

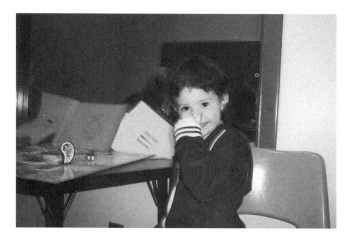

Figure 4-4 ■ Client with phoneme-specific nasal emission is occluding her nostrils while practicing production of /s/ tokens.

Research Note   A mirror used to observe articulatory placements and diagrams of those articulators can provide helpful performance feedback for clients.

Trost-Cardamone, 1990a.

The **See Scape** (Pro-Ed, Austin, Tex.) is a commercially made device that can also be used for feedback purposes. It consists of tubing attached to a glass piston. The glass piston contains a small piece of Styrofoam that is sensitive to airflow. A nasal olive connected to the tubing is placed in contact with one naris; any unwanted nasal air pressure can then be detected by displacement of the Styrofoam within the piston. The See Scape can also be used to provide visual feedback of oral pressure. In this case the nasal olive can be placed between the lips, and the release of the oral air pressure for production of speech sounds such as the plosives /p, b/ is present visually for the client. A **water manometer** is a device used to measure air pressure; it can also be used similarly to the See Scape to identify either oral air pressure or nasal air pressure. Drinking straws may also be used in the same manner. When placed between the lips, the oral release of air into the straw creates an auditory percept that may assist the child in developing an oral focus. One additional feedback tool is an air paddle—a small strip of paper that is held under the client's nose when producing oral practice material. If unwanted nasal emission occurs, then the air paddle shows movement. The reader should also note that sophisticated instrumentation such as aerodynamic equipment (Peterson-Falzone et al., 2001) can be used for feedback purposes; however, many practitioners do not have access to such equipment because they do not have substantial numbers of clients with cleft palate.

Sound System Error Treatment Specifics

The rationale for introducing /h/ is to have the patient produce a speech sound that is not physiologically compatible with glottal stop production. Introducing /h/ and incorporating the speech sound in a core of syllables and then words that can be practiced by the child is an important first step in eliminating compensatory articulations. Generally the client can imitate a model produced by the clinician, and the model can be prolonged to approximate a whisper. Once correct production is achieved, the target sound is incorporated into different word positions (prevocalic and intervocalic positions) and levels of practice such as syllables, words, phrases, and sentences. For example, the clinician may initially want to introduce practice with the /h/ in the prevocalic position at the syllable level. When the client has met the appropriate response accuracy criterion, practice shifts to a different word position or level of practice material, such as phrases, sentences, and conversations.

In addition to breaking the glottal stop pattern, achievement of correct /h/ production can also be used as a coarticulating sound for the introduction of other sounds. That is, the clinician can use the sound as a basis for producing other sounds that are misarticulated. Golding-Kushner (2001) also recommends the use of imagery to create a distinction between the error sound and the target sound. For example, the clinician may want to designate a glottal stop production as a *coughing sound* and the target sound as a *mouth sound* or *breezy sound*. These designations are designed to help the child develop a perception of the intended target and help break up the posterior articulation pattern. The clinician identifies correct productions and errors, and the appropriate feedback is given to the client. For example, "No, you made the coughing sound. I need you to make the /p/ popping sound."

Research Note	The use of imagery may be helpful in the treatment of sound system errors to create a distinction between the error sound and the target sound.

Golding-Kushner, 2001.

After the achievement of correct /h/ production, treatment shifts to the sound groups listed in Table 4-2. The first group of sounds includes the **bilabials** /m, p, b/. Generally the child produces nasals, but if the /m/ is not in the child's inventory, it needs to be taught. One technique is to instruct the child to close the lips and hum a song (Golding-Kushner, 2001). This technique will often result in the production of /m/.

The other sounds in this group are the **plosive cognates** /p, b/. These sounds are pressure sounds and require the generation of satisfactory intraoral air pressure. A glottal stop substitution is frequently used in place of the bilabial productions. When working with cognates, the voiceless sound should be introduced first. Golding-Kushner (2001) suggests that the clinician have the client prolong /h/ and then close and open the lips to produce the /p/ sound. With some clients the nostrils must be occluded to prevent air from escaping through the nose. Some of the other feedback techniques that were summarized may also be used to emphasize an oral focus or identify unwanted nasal emission. The aim is to create the explosion or release of air for the plosive by air impounded behind the lips. Kummer (2001b) recommends that the client be taught to whisper the /p/ with the adjacent vowel, because whisper will prevent vocal fold adduction. Another technique advocated by Riski (2006) is to instruct the client to puff out the cheeks and make the /p/ sound. Correct production of the cognate /b/ may be elicited by instructing the client to make the sound like /p/ but turn on the voice (or have the client produce an /m/ and then occlude the nostrils to achieve articulation of /b/). Once production is achieved, the target sound is then incorporated into different word positions and levels of practice material as discussed previously.

In the treatment of the bilabial plosive cognates, the aim is to increase the explosion or release of air for the plosive by air impounded behind the lips. The client may be taught to whisper the /p/ with the adjacent vowel, because a whisper will prevent vocal fold adduction. Another technique is to instruct the client to puff out the cheeks and make the /p/ sound.

Research Note

Kummer, 2001b; Riski, 2006.

After introducing the bilabials, the **labiodental fricatives** /f, v/ are then targeted. Oftentimes, children will substitute a pharyngeal fricative in place of the target sounds. The child should be instructed to prolong the /h/ and then bring the lower lip and upper teeth together to produce the target sound. Golding-Kuhsner (2001) cautions against instructing the client with the verbal cue "bite the lip," because this may result in a restricted constriction of the lip and teeth. While the client produces the sound, the clinician digitally occludes the client's nostrils because air is typically channeled through the nasal tract during the initial stages of treatment. When the client is able to direct the airstream orally and use the correct point of articulation, digital occlusion may be eliminated. The voiced cognate /v/ is taught by having the client superimpose voicing with the labiodental production. Verbal imagery cues such as "buzz like a bee, or make a humming sound" can be used to facilitate voicing. Occlusion of the nostrils is also used with the voiced cognate, if necessary.

In the treatment of labiodental fricatives, the client should prolong the /h/ sound and bring the lower lip and upper teeth together to produce the target sound. The clinician should avoid instructing the client with the verbal cue "bite the lip," because this instruction may result in a restricted constriction of the lip and teeth.

Research Note

Golding-Kushner, 2001.

The next suggested group of sounds to be taught are those that involve linguadental and alveolar articulations. The fricative pair /θ, ð/ are visible sounds that are taught in the same manner as the labiodental fricatives, but the placement cues will differ. The client is typically instructed to "place the tongue tip between the teeth and make the air come out your mouth." Occluding the nostrils, or other feedback techniques, may be used during the initial teaching of the target sounds if necessary. Golding-Kushner (2001) points out that /θ, ð/ may serve as facilitating sounds for the fricatives /s, z/, so correct placement can aid in the introduction of other pressure sounds. The lingua-alveolar sounds /n, t, d/ are then introduced if the child does not articulate the sounds correctly. Initially, the nasal /n/ is taught. The child is instructed, "Open your mouth a little and touch your tongue behind your upper teeth. Once you touch, you need to let your tongue go." The child should also be informed that /n/ is like /m/; consequently, sound energy will come from the nose. The plosives /t, d/ follow the introduction of /n/. Golding-Kushner (2001) recommends that the sound elicitation technique used for /p, b/ also be used for /t, d/ because they are also plosive sounds. That is, the client is instructed to prolong the /h/ and alternately contact and release the tongue tip as it creates a constriction with the alveolar ridge. The technique can be modeled for the child so that he or she is given appropriate auditory and visual information requisite to production (/hhhhhhhtʌ/). If the plosives are produced as middorsum palatal stops, then the place of articulation needs to be shifted forward to the alveolar point of articulation. Placement information, including diagrams and models, can be useful in developing the appropriate place or articulation.

The **alveolar fricatives** /s, z/ are frequently problematic for children with cleft palate, and initial work should be carried out with the nostrils occluded. Riski (2006) has proposed a number of teaching strategies for acquiring correct production in isolation. One strategy is to have the client produce the /θ/ and then move the tongue behind the front teeth to approximate /s/ placement. The client can be cued in the following way: "Make the /θ/; keep making it and slide your tongue just behind your teeth. Listen for the difference in the sound when your tongue goes behind your teeth." Another strategy is to have the child produce /t/ and then release the sound to make an /s/, or the child can be instructed to repeat /t/ and transition to an /s/ production /ttttt sssss/. Golding-Kushner (2001) suggests that a word with the /t/ in the postvocalic position be used to elicit /s/. The client is stimulated to produce a word such as /pɛ t/ and instructed to prolong the /t/ at the end of the word. This strategy often results in the target production /pɛts/. The /z/ can be obtained by cuing the client to produce a sustained /s/ and then "turn on the speech motor" so that /z/ is articulated /sssssszzzzzz/. Correct production of the alveolar fricatives is an important achievement for the child with cleft lip and palate.

The next set of sounds are the **velars** /ŋ, k, g/. According to Golding-Kushner (1995), some clients may have difficulty in acquiring correct production of the velar plosives /k, g/ because their placement is most posterior in the vocal tract and intended productions may trigger pharyngeal or glottal stop substitutions. In some cases clients will produce the stops anteriorly as middorsum palatal stops. Peterson-Falzone and colleagues (2006) indicate that the production of middorsum stops blurs the perceptual boundaries between alveolar and velar stops. Listeners may have difficulty discriminating /t-k/ and /d-g/. Consequently, it is recommended that the nasal /ŋ/ be introduced initially. The reader should note that /ŋ/ occurs in the intervocalic and postvocalic word positions; it does not occur in the prevocalic position. A coarticulation technique for /ŋ/ is to have the client produce the sound in the intervocalic position using the vowel /i/ as a juxtaposed sound (/iŋi/). Golding-Kushner (2001) feels that the vowel coarticulatory context minimizes the probability of triggering a more posterior articulation because the vowel articulation involves a high front tongue position. When correct production of /ŋ/ is achieved, the nasal can be used in a facilitating way to achieve production of the voiced velar plosive /g/. To achieve production of /g/, the client can be instructed to "make the sound with the back of the tongue, and make it a longer sound while I hold your nose." The clinician can then provide an imitative model of the sequence /iŋgi-iŋgi-iŋgi/ for the child to repeat. This contextual stimulus is then followed by the child's repetition with the nostrils occluded. Correct production is followed by a transition to the coarticulatory stimulus /iŋgi-gi/ with the nostrils occluded. Once the /g/ productions are achieved, practice will shift to syllable or word stimuli without occluding the nostrils. The /k/ is then introduced and the child is cued: "Make the /g/ sound, but don't turn on your voice motor. Just let the air come out when you make the sound." The voiced plosive sound is taught first, rather than the typical voiceless–voiced sequence that has been followed. The reason for this alteration is a clinical hypothesis that children with cleft palate have less difficulty acquiring /g/, and the /ŋ/ is a facilitating coarticulatory influence for /g/.

Research Note	Some clients have difficulty acquiring correct production of the velar plosives /k, g/ because the correct placement of these sounds is most posterior in the vocal tract and intended productions may trigger middorsum pharyngeal or glottal stop substitutions.

Golding-Kushner, 1995.

The final set of sounds in the sequence are the **palatal fricatives** /ʃ, ʒ/ and affricates /tʃ, dʒ/. These sounds are also pressure sounds and are frequently misarticulated by children with clefts. Some techniques for eliciting /ʃ/ include instructing the child to "pull the tongue back a little bit when you make /s/ so that you make /ʃ/." The movement from /s/ to /ʃ/ is often a facilitating context for some clients (Riski, 2006). If needed, the child's nostrils can be occluded to facilitate appropriate air pressure buildup. Kummer (2001b) recommends that the client be instructed to produce a "big sigh" with the teeth closed and lips rounded. The client can use the technique while being cued to "move the tongue until you make the whisper sound /ʃ/." Voicing cues such as "turn on your motor and make the sound /ʒ/" can be used after correct placement of /ʃ/. As with the /ʃ/, it may be necessary to occlude the nostrils with /ʒ/. Incorporation of /ʒ/ in words will be in the intervocalic and postvocalic word positions. Affricates combine the production features of both stops and fricatives. A complete occlusion of the vocal tract occurs, followed by a sustained release. One facilitating technique is to have the client produce /t t t t t/ and then shift the tongue tip to the palatal point of articulation and make /tʃ/. Another sound elicitation technique is to instruct the child to sneeze by starting with the mouth closed and then producing the /tʃ/ (Kummer, 2001b). The voiced cognate /dʒ/ can be shaped in the same way as discussed with /ʒ/. A summary of the treatment components is listed in Box 4-3.

Research Note	Correct placement of palatal fricatives may be achieved by instructing the client to produce a "big sigh" with the teeth closed and the lips rounded while moving the tongue until the client can make a whisper sound /ʃ/.

Kummer, 2001b.

> **BOX 4-3** *Treatment Components for Children with Cleft Lip and Palate*
>
> - Different types of feedback are necessary to create an awareness of the production features of the error versus the target sound.
> - The clinician should introduce verbal imagery to create an internal contrast between the error sound and the target sound.
> - Treatment of sounds should begin with /h/ if necessary, with subsequent target sounds introduced from an anterior to a posterior placement progression.
> - Sound facilitation techniques are used to develop the appropriate voice, place, and manner features of target sounds.

Additional Treatment Concerns

The reader should note that many children with cleft palate frequently produce lingual fricatives and affricates in a lateralized manner. Trost-Cardamone (1990b) suggests that a client with cleft lip and palate who has a lateral crossbite (see Dental and Occlusal Problems) may exhibit lateralization of lingual fricatives, affricates, or both. Lateralization is a nondevelopmental oral articulation distortion that involves directing the airstream off the sides of the tongue, rather than using a central airstream. However, this type of error is also found in the articulation of clients without velopharyngeal closure deficits.

Clinicians should note that lateralization in the presence of the malocclusion may be an obligatory error caused by an existing dental condition. However, because this author is not aware of any literature demonstrating the spontaneous elimination of lateralization with dental or orthodontic correction of an existing malocclusion, therapy is necessary to correct the problem. Riski (2006) recommends the release of /t/ to /s/ as described previously. Some practitioners also recommend the use of coarticulatory facilitation to elicit a target sound. For example, the client may be asked to repeat the phrase "get you" and then be instructed to gradually blend the two words together so that the result is /tʃ/.

The oral semivowels /w, j, l, r/ are not discussed in terms of specific teaching techniques because the sounds are voiced open sounds and do not require the generation of oral pressure. The sounds may be produced with hypernasal resonance, but Trost-Cardamone (1990a) indicated that the /l, r/ speech sounds are sometimes produced at a velar point of articulation by some clients with cleft palate—the /l/ → /L/ and the /r/ → /R/. The practitioner should be alert to the possibility that the sounds may be produced with a more posterior point of articulation; however, the backing of the two semivowels is also seen in the speech of clients without velopharyngeal closure deficits. If identified, the errors should be treated.

Other Structural Deficits: Treatment Considerations

Following is a discussion of other structural deficits that the practitioner may encounter. These structural variants may or may not be causal factors in the development and maintenance of a speech sound disorder. Moreover, if they are determined to be causal factors, then the problems are generally associated with obligatory errors that require treatment from different dental and medical specialties. Trost-Cardamone (1990b) cautions that research is limited regarding structural deficits and their effect on speech sound production; consequently, any guidelines "should be applied flexibly and thoughtfully." The role of the speech-language pathologist will vary but should always include the client's caregivers; they must be informed so that they can make the appropriate decision regarding management of the child. In some instances the practitioner is also the referral agent, and in others he or she is a consultant who provides information to other professionals regarding the potential effects of the structural problem on communication and feeding. In either case the practitioner should evaluate the child's speech production skills before and after dental and medical treatment and determine whether communication intervention is necessary.

Lingual Problems

The tongue is a key oral structure for speech production and the act of swallowing (Daniloff, 1973; Logemann, 1998; Perkins and Kent, 1986; Perlman and Christensen, 1997). Kier and Smith (1985) characterize the tongue as a *muscular hydrostat*; as such, it does not have primary skeletal support. The key feature of a muscular hydrostat is that it is capable of assuming different shapes without changing its volume. Intrinsic and extrinsic muscles play major roles in support and movement of the tongue. Anatomically, the tongue is divided into the tip, blade, dorsum, and root or tongue base (Daniloff, 1973). Generally most tongue growth takes place by 8 years of age, and very little growth is expected after 12 years of age.

> The tongue is characterized as a *muscular hydrostat*; as such, it does not have primary skeletal support. The key feature of a muscular hydrostat is that it is capable of assuming different shapes without changing its volume.
>
> *Research Note*

Kier and Smith, 1985.

Relative judgments of tongue size are problematic for the speech-language pathologist because the tongue is situated in the oral cavity space and bounded by the maxilla and mandible. **Macroglossia** describes an unusually large tongue, whereas **hypoglossia** is a term used to describe an abnormally small tongue. A tongue that seems unusually large may actually be normal in mass if the mandible or lower jaw is limited in size, as seen in cases of Pierre Robin Sequence (Shprintzen, 1997). Shprintzen and Witzel (1993) indicate that malformations of the tongue occur less frequently than anomalies of the palate; however, some syndromes include characteristics such as tongue anomalies. For example, macroglossia is often associated with **Beckwith-Wiedemann syndrome,** and hypoglossia is frequently found in individuals with **hypoglossia-hypodactyly sequence.** Clefting of the tongue or lobulation is a condition found infrequently; however, the condition is associated with a number of syndromes such as **oral-facial-digital syndrome, type I** (Jung, 1989; Shprintzen, 1997, 2000; Shprintzen and Bardach, 1995).

Gasparini and colleagues (2002) indicate that markers of macroglossia are protrusion of the tip and blade of the tongue beyond the dental arch during resting posture, dental marks on the lingual margins of the tongue, or both. The seminal work of Van Borsel and colleagues (2000) was the first to analyze and carefully describe the articulatory patterns of children with macroglossia. The authors indicated that the most frequent errors were consonant productions with a more anterior point of articulation. The predominant error type was distortion, and distortions were found for bilabial, labiodental, alveolar, and palatal points of articulation (Figure 4-5). For example, bilabial sounds are made with the upper and lower lips in contact with the protruding tongue, rather than exclusive bilabial contact. Tongue-tip alveolar sounds such as /s, z, t, d, n, l/ are produced as blade alveolar sounds. In summary, manner is preserved; however, the point of articulation is anterior to the regular point of articulation.

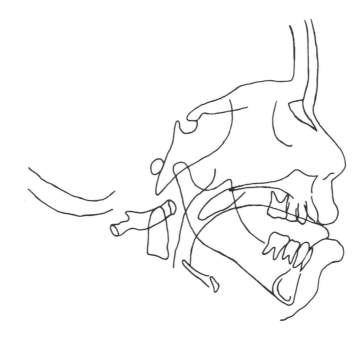

Figure 4-5 ■ Lateral-view cephalometric tracing of a young client with macroglossia producing /s/ in isolation. Note the forward tongue position, with the tongue tip protruding between the lips.

Research Note	Markers of macroglossia have been identified as (1) protrusion of the tip and blade of the tongue beyond the dental arch during resting posture and/or (2) dental marks on the lingual margins of the tongue.

Gasparini et al., 2002.

Murthy and Laing (1994) indicate that an interdisciplinary team approach to management is necessary and needs to include the speech-language pathologist along with the appropriate medical and dental specialists. Initial concerns for some infants with macroglossia are airway compromise and the possibility of dysphagia, including problems with saliva control. Evaluation is necessary to determine the status of respiration and oral-feeding skills. If problems are detected, then the speech-language pathologist will need to make management recommendations in consultation with medical personnel. In addition, the parents will need information from the team regarding the presenting problems, recommended interventions, and potential problems that the child may face in the future. Support groups for children with special needs such as Beckwith-Wiedemann syndrome are available and of great assistance to parents (Weng et al., 1995).

As the child develops, speech, tongue resting posture, and dentoskeletal growth are variables that the interdisciplinary team must observe carefully. In some cases, counseling services may also be needed because of aesthetic concerns of the client and family. The speech-language pathologist will need to evaluate speech and tongue resting posture, and the medical and dental specialists will need to monitor dentoskeletal growth. After the assessments, treatment plans that include caregiver input will need to be developed for the child. In many cases the treatment plan will include a tongue resection, because an enlarged tongue negatively influences dentoskeletal growth. When surgical intervention is recommended, the speech-language pathologist must carry out baseline assessments of articulation and tongue resting posture for postoperative comparison. After recovery from surgery, treatment for articulation may be necessary because the anatomy and physiology of tongue has been modified.

Case studies of children with hypoglossia generally report that the lower jaw or mandible is also reduced in size (Peterson-Falzone, 1988). The smaller size of the mandible is known as *micrognathia*. Descriptions of speech production skills typically indicate that individuals with hypoglossia develop intelligible speech.

Ankyloglossia, or tongue-tie, is a condition that occurs on an infrequent basis, but a speech-language pathologist may see children with the problem (Lalakea and Messner, 2003). The condition may or may not be problematic for a specific client and is found more frequently in males than females (approximate ratio, 3:1). The presence of the condition does not mean that a definite problem exists. Although it occurs most often as an isolated anatomic variation, a higher prevalence has been found in infants with a history of maternal cocaine use and certain birth syndromes such as **Optiz syndrome,** orodigitofacial syndrome, and in combination with **X-linked cleft palate.** In some limited cases, ankyloglossia has been found to be problematic in breastfeeding; however, no problems have been reported in the case of bottle-feeding or solid foods.

The literature suggests that individuals with ankyloglossia that adversely affects speech production skills may demonstrate difficulty in producing the lingua-alveolar speech sounds (/t, d, s, z, n, l/) (Lalakea and Messner, 2003). In addition, older children and adults with ankyloglossia often complain of difficulty performing some mechanical fuctions such as clearing the lips, playing a woodwind instrument, and kissing. The diagnosis of ankyloglossia is a frenum that is attached at or near the tip of the tongue, which is hypothesized to restrict the movements of the tongue. When the tongue is protruded, it may exhibit a heart-shaped appearance with the inversion at midline because of the restricted frenum. Although no definitive data exist, some individuals measure such variables as tongue protrusion, interincisal distance, and other lingual dimensions (Fletcher and Meldrum, 1968; Williams and Waldron, 1985). Range of lingual protrusion is studied by having the client stick out the tongue and measuring the underside distance from the tongue tip to the blade of the tongue at the outer surface of the lower incisor teeth. Interincisal distance is the distance between the upper and lower incisors when the client places the tongue tip at the back posterior edge of the upper central incisors and the mouth is open completely. In both measurements, Lalakea and Messner (2003) have found values in the range of 15 mm or less for patients with ankyloglossia and 20 to 25 mm or greater for normal patients. The speech-language pathologist can use the measurement procedure and must also consider speech sound production skills and any accompanying problems, if present. If no speech sound problems (particularly the lingua-alveolar sounds) or complaints concerning other lingual functions exist, then surgical release of the frenum is not warranted.

Research Note	Research suggests that individuals with ankyloglossia that adversely affects speech production skills may have difficulty producing the lingua-alveolar speech sounds (/t, d, s, z, n, l/).

Lalakea and Messner, 2003.

Research Note	Interincisal distance is the space between the upper and lower incisors when the patient places his or her tongue tip at the back posterior edge of the upper central incisors while the mouth is open completely. Researchers have found values in the range of 15 mm or less for individuals with ankyloglossia and 20 to 25 mm or more for individuals who do not exhibit this lingual problem.

Lalakea and Messner, 2003.

CASE STUDY 4-2

Obligatory Errors: Postponement of Treatment

S.U. received a diagnosis of macroglossia at birth and was first seen for a speech and language evaluation at age 3 years, 6 months. A speech-language pathologist who had seen the child at a local preschool program referred her to the clinic for further assessment. Intake history indicated that the client had speech sound production errors and displayed a habitual open-mouth resting posture with tongue protrusion. The child's mother indicated that overall developmental history was generally uneventful. She was concerned about speech development and resting tongue posture. According to S.U.'s mother, the child's tongue appeared very large at birth and protruded from the mouth, but the size of the tongue and its protrusion did not interfere with either feeding or sleeping. The child had undergone various medical diagnostic procedures, including a genetics evaluation, which failed to identify a cause of the macroglossia.

Sound production skills were examined through administration of an articulation test and spontaneous conversational sample. Bilabial, labiodental, linguadental, alveolar, and palatal consonant speech sounds were judged to be misarticulated. The child preserved the manner of articulation and the voice and voiceless features, but place of articulation was not maintained because of the macroglossia and obligatory tongue protrusion. Bilabial sounds /p, b, m/ were articulated as linguolabial sounds. The linguadental fricatives /θ,ð/ were produced at the appropriate place of articulation, but the blade (and not the tip) was used to make dental contact. Alveolar and palatal sounds /t, d, n, l, s, z, ʃ, ʒ, tʃ, dʒ/ were made as blade linguadental sounds; the blade was in contact with the upper teeth. The velar plosives /k, g/ were judged as being correctly articulated. An additional sound system error that appeared developmental was /j/ in substitution of /r/ in prevocalic and intervocalic word positions.

Sound system errors of deletion, which are frequently used by young clients, were not identified during the testing. The error pattern appeared to be motor- or phonetic-based rather than phonologically based. S.U. was maintaining the manner of articulation, but obligatory tongue placement resulted in the perceptual judgment of distortion errors. Phonotactically, S.U. used both simple and complex syllable shapes spontaneously and in the context of testing.

A test of word intelligibility was administered and audiotaped to obtain an estimate of the subject's intelligibility. The tape was evaluated by two student clinicians unfamiliar with the client, and a mean intelligibility rating of 74% was found. The results suggested that intelligibility at the single-word level was only moderately impaired. Stimulability testing was initiated, but S.U. would not imitate the target stimuli. Expressive and receptive language were screened and found to be within normal limits. S.U. also passed a hearing screening for pure tones.

An oral examination was carried out to examine the structure and function of the speech mechanism. S.U. was in the primary dentition stage and exhibited a Class III occlusion with an anterior open bite. That is, the lower jaw or mandible extended slightly beyond the upper jaw or maxilla. An opening also existed between the upper and lower front teeth when the upper and lower molars were in contact. At rest position the tongue protruded from the oral cavity. The blade rested on the lower lip, and the tip extended slightly beyond the lower lip. Even though the client showed a habitual open-mouth posture, drooling was not observed during the oral examination.

After the speech and language evaluation, an interdisciplinary consultation with a pediatric dentist, orthodontist, oral surgeon, speech-language pathologist, and S.U.'s parents was arranged. The dental specialists corroborated the open-mouth/tongue protrusion resting posture, Class III occlusion, and anterior open bite. The orthodontist indicated that the tongue position and open-mouth posture was not conducive to dental occlusion and the eventual eruption of the permanent teeth. A tongue resection was also discussed, because generally this is a part of the treatment for clients with macroglossia.

Commentary

Treatment for the sound system disorder is contraindicated because the sound errors that were identified are obligatory. The client has a macroglossia and open bite. These structural conditions prevent appropriate placement of bilabials, labiodentals, linguadentals, alveolars, and palatal sounds. An interdisciplinary treatment plan with the appropriate professionals was needed for S.U. because of the complex structural conditions. When the structural conditions have been corrected, the speech-language pathologist should carry out a reevaluation to determine whether treatment is necessary. The course of treatment for S.U. is a tongue resection, correction of the alignment of the upper and lower jaw, and correction of the open bite. The reader should note that in many cases a change in structure results in a positive change in function. That is, the client may not require speech treatment if the structural condition has been eliminated, because correction of oral structural form may facilitate correct placement of sounds that were in error.

Dental and Occlusal Problems

When examining dentition, the practitioner may see children with missing teeth, rotated teeth, or teeth that are not in proper position, and he or she must determine whether the speech disorder is caused by the presenting dental condition (St. Louis and Ruscello, 2000). A review by Bernthal and Bankson (2004) indicates that rotated or supernumerary (extra) teeth typically do not affect speech production skills; however, missing teeth may influence articulation skills. That is, in some cases, missing teeth, particularly the upper central and lateral incisors, may affect the production of the labiodental, linguadental, and lingua-alveolar fricatives differently; however, the practitioner must remember that many clients exhibit such structural problems in the presence of normal sound production skills. The potential effect must be evaluated on a case-by-case basis.

The clinician needs to evaluate individually the potential effect of different dental conditions on speech.

Research Note

Bernthal and Bankson, 2004.

Open bite is the presence of a gap or opening between the anterior maxillary and mandibular teeth (Peterson-Falzone et al., 2001). Researchers have hypothesized that an open bite is a function of consistent mouth breathing or thumb sucking. Although the practitioner is probably familiar with an anterior open bite, he or she may also see clients with lateral open bite. This is a dental condition of spacing between the maxillary and mandibular molars and bicuspids (Figure 4-6). Lingual protrusion or lisping of /s, z/ may be present in clients who have an anterior open bite. Trost-Cardamone (1990b) indicates that lateralization may be seen in clients with lateral open bites. A **crossbite** is another condition wherein the maxillary teeth are shifted and lingual to the mandibular teeth (Peterson-Falzone et al., 2001; Figure 4-7). A client with an anterior crossbite may demonstrate a problem that ranges from an individual upper incisor that is shifted behind the corresponding lower incisor to all the incisors behind or distal to the lower incisors. A buccal or lateral crossbite is a lateral shifting of the teeth that are situated near the buccal cavity or cheeks. A client may exhibit unilateral or bilateral involvement.

Peterson-Falzone (1988) writes that an anterior crossbite may be associated with misarticulations of lingua-alveolar sounds, because the

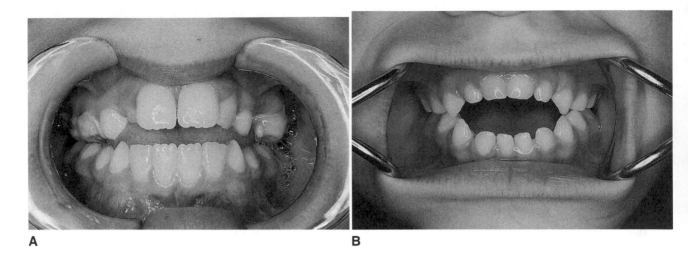

A   B

Figure 4-6 ■ Two individuals with anterior open bites with different degrees of severity. (From Peterson-Falzone SJ, Hardin-Jones MA, Karnell MP: *Cleft palate speech*, ed 3, St Louis, 2001, Mosby.)

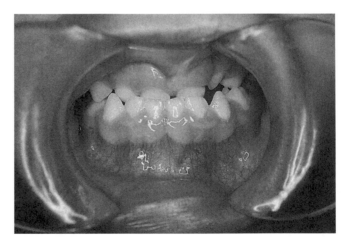

Figure 4-7 ■ Individual with an anterior crossbite. (From Peterson-Falzone SJ, Hardin-Jones MA, Karnell MP: *Cleft palate speech*, ed 3, St Louis, 2001, Mosby.)

alveolus is shifted posteriorly as a result of mandibular overlap, thus affecting the normal relationship with the tongue. A buccal or lateral crossbite may be conducive to the development of lateralization (as discussed in the treatment of clients with cleft lip and palate).

There is a likelihood of misarticulation of lingua-alveolar sounds in the case of an anterior crossbite.	*Research Note*

Peterson-Falzone, 1988.

Dental occlusion is the relationship of the upper dental arch (maxilla) to the lower dental arch (mandible) (Zemlin, 1998). In normal occlusion (Class I), the cusps of the mandibular first molar and maxillary first molar are in contact; the mandibular molar is a half cusp ahead and inside the maxillary first molar. A Class I malocclusion includes a normal molar relationship, but some anterior dental variation is seen. In a Class II malocclusion, the cusps of the mandibular molars are behind and inside the maxillary molars. The upper dental arch is shifted forward or ahead of the lower arch. The Class II condition is most frequently found in clients with malocclusion. When the mandibular first molar is ahead of the maxillary first molar, a Class III malocclusion is present. The lower jaw is shifted forward with respect to the upper jaw, and the client shows a prominent chin. Class II malocclusion has been associated with /s/ production errors; in some cases clients were reported to have difficulty achieving lip closure for bilabial sounds. Bilabial, labiodental, and alveolar points of articulation can be problematic for speakers with a Class III malocclusion, because the lower jaw is ahead of the upper jaw. Figure 4-8 illustrates normal occlusion and malocclusions according to Angle's classification.

A review of the literature by Peterson-Falzone (1988) indicates that different structural conditions such as missing, crooked, or malpositioned teeth and open bite or crossbite may or may not influence a client's articulation. A Class II malocclusion may be associated with placement errors, particularly if the malocclusion is a severe expression; placement errors are frequently found in the speech of clients with Class III malocclusion. When clients undergo dental, orthodontic, or surgical procedures, changes in structural form frequently facilitate changes in speech function (Corcoran, 2001).

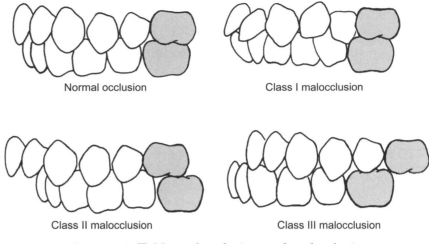

Normal occlusion

Class I malocclusion

Class II malocclusion

Class III malocclusion

Figure 4-8 ■ Normal occlusion and malocclusion classes according to Angle's classification. (From Proffit WR: *Contemporary orthodontics,* ed 3, St Louis, 2000, Mosby.)

SUMMARY

A small subset of clients has sound system errors and coexisting structural deficits. The structural problems can range from a missing tooth to a complete cleft of the lip and palate. For these individuals, categorizing their sound system errors as *developmental, obligatory,* or *compensatory* is useful. Developmental errors are not related to an oral structural deficit; a client may spontaneously acquire the sounds or receive treatment if they are not acquired within the expected developmental period. Obligatory errors are related to a structural deficit and generally do not respond to behavioral speech treatment. They are frequently produced as distortions of the intended target. If obligatory errors are present, then referral to dental and medical specialists may be necessary to correct the structural problem. Compensatory errors are also found in the speech of children with structural deficits and used in substitution of a sound or an entire sound class. Specific techniques from a motor skill–learning perspective are described to remediate compensatory errors in clients with cleft lip and palate. Additional structural deficits are discussed, and recommendations concerning management are summarized for the clinician.

REFERENCES

Bernthal JE, Bankson NW: *Articulation and phonological disorders,* ed 5, Boston, 2004, Allyn & Bacon.

Chapman K: Phonologic processes in children with cleft palate, *Cleft Palate Craniofac J* 30:64-71, 1993.

Corcoran J: Orthognathic surgery for craniofacial differences. In Kummer AW, editor: *Cleft palate and craniofacial anomalies: the effects of speech and resonance,* San Diego, 2001, Singular.

Daniloff RG: Normal articulation processes. In Minifie FD, Hixon TJ, Williams F, editors: *Normal aspects of speech, hearing, and language,* Englewood Cliffs, NJ, 1973, Prentice-Hall.

Fletcher SC, Meldrum JR: Lingual function and relative length of the lingual frenulum, *J Speech Hear Res* 11:382-390, 1968.

Gasparini G, Saltarel A, Carboni A et al: Surgical management of macroglossia: discussion of 7 cases, *Surg Pathol Oral Radiol* 94:566-571, 2002.

Gibbon FE, Crampin L: An electropalatographic investigation of middorsum palatal stops in an adult with repaired cleft palate, *Cleft Palate Craniofac J* 38:96-105, 2001.

Golding-Kushner KJ: Treatment of articulation and resonance disorders associated with cleft palate and VPI. In Shprintzen RJ, Bardach J, editors: *Cleft palate speech management: a multidisciplinary approach,* St Louis, 1995, Mosby.

Golding-Kushner KJ: *Therapy techniques for cleft palate speech and related disorders,* San Diego, 2001, Singular.

Golding-Kushner KJ: Treatment of sound system disorders associated with cleft palate speech, *SID 5 Newsletter* 14:16-19, 2004.

Crames T M· Implementing treatment recommendations: role of the craniofacial team speech-language pathologist in working with the client's speech-language pathologist, *SID 5 Newsletter* 14:6-9, 2004.

Hardin-Jones MA, Jones DL: Speech production of preschoolers with cleft palate, *Cleft Palate Craniofac J* 42:7-13, 2005.

Henningsson GE, Isberg AM: Velopharyngeal movements in patients alternating between oral and glottal articulation: a clinical and cineradiographical study, *Cleft Palate J* 23:1-9, 1986.

Jung JH: *Genetic syndromes in communicative disorders,* Boston, 1989, College-Hill Press.

Kier WM, Smith KK: Tongues, tentacles and trunks: the biomechanics of movement in muscular-hydrostats, *Zool J Linn Soc* 83:307-324, 1985.

Kuehn DP, Moller KT: Speech and language issues in the cleft palate population: the state of the art, *Cleft Palate Craniofac J* 37:348-1-348-35, 2000.

Kummer AW: Perceptual assessment. In Kummer AW, editor: *Cleft palate and craniofacial anomalies: the effects of speech and resonance,* San Diego, 2001a, Singular.

Kummer AW: Speech therapy for effects of velopharyngeal dysfunction. In Kummer AW, editor: *Cleft palate and craniofacial anomalies: the effects of speech and resonance,* San Diego, 2001b, Singular.

Kummer AW, Strife JL, Grau WH et al: The effects of Le Fort I osteotomy with maxillary advancement on articulation, resonance, and velopharyngeal function, *Cleft Palate J* 26:193-199, 1989.

Lalakea ML, Messner AH: Ankyloglossia: does it matter? *Pediatr Clin North Am* 50:381-397, 2003.

Logemann JA: *Evaluation and treatment of swallowing disorders,* ed 2, Austin, Tex, 1998, Pro-Ed.

Marino VCC, Williams WN, Wharton PW et al: Immediate and sustained changes in tongue movement with an experimental palatal "fistula": a case study, *Cleft Palate Craniofac J* 42:286-296, 2005.

McWilliams BJ, Morris HL, Shelton RL: *Cleft palate speech,* Philadelphia, 1984, BC Decker.

Miccio AW: A treatment program for enhancing stimulability. In Kamhi AG, Pollock KE, editors: *Phonological disorders in children,* Baltimore, 2005, Paul H Brookes.

Moller KT: Dental-occlusal and other oral conditions and speech. In Bernthal J, Bankson N, editors: *Child phonology: characteristics, assessment, and intervention in special populations,* New York, 1994, Thieme Medical.

Morris HL: Some questions and answers about velopharyngeal dysfunction during speech, *Am J Speech Lang Pathol* 1:26-28, 1992.

Murthy P, Laing MR: Macroglossia, *Br Med J* 26:1386-1387, 1994.

Pamplona M, Ysunza A: A comparative trial of two modalities of speech intervention cleft palate children: phonologic vs. articulatory approach, *Int J Pediatr Otorhinolaryngol* 49:2-27, 1999.

Perkins WH, Kent RD: *Functional anatomy of speech, language, and hearing,* San Diego, 1986, College-Hill Press.

Perlman AL, Christensen J: Topography and functional anatomy of the swallowing structures. In Perlman AD, Schulze-Delrieu D, editors: *Deglutition and its measurement,* San Diego, 1997, Singular.

Peterson-Falzone SJ: Speech disorders related to craniofacial structural defects. In Lass NJ, McReynolds LV, Northern JL et al, editors: *Handbook of speech-language pathology and audiology,* Philadelphia, 1988, BC Decker.

Peterson-Falzone SJ, Hardin-Jones MA, Karnell M: *Cleft palate speech,* ed 3, St Louis, 2001, Mosby.

Peterson-Falzone SJ, Trost-Cardamone JE, Karnell M et al: *The clinician's guide to treating cleft palate speech,* St Louis, 2006, Mosby.

Proffit WR: *Contemporary orthodontics,* ed 3, St Louis, 2000, Mosby.

Riski JE: *Managing speech disorders: improving your clinical competence with articulation disorders related to cleft lip/palate and craniofacial disorders,* Atlanta, 2006, Children's Healthcare of Atlanta. Available at: www.choa.org/default.aspx?id = 761. Accessed November 8, 2006.

Ruscello DM: The oral examination. In Ruscello DM, editor: *Tests and measurements in speech-language pathology,* Boston, 2001, Butterworth-Heinemann.

Ruscello DM: Residual phonological errors. In Kent R, editor: *Encyclopedia of communication disorders,* Boston, 2003, MIT Press.

Ruscello DM: Considerations for behavioral treatment of velopharyngeal closure for speech. In Bzoch K, editor: *Communicative disorders related to cleft lip and palate,* ed 5, Austin, Tex, 2004, Pro-Ed.

Ruscello DM, Douglas C, Tyson T et al: Macroglossia: a case study, *J Commun Disord* 38: 109-122, 2005.

Ruscello DM, Tekieli ME, Van Sickels JE: Speech production before and after orthognathic surgery: a review, *Oral Surg Oral Med Oral Pathol* 59: 10-14, 1985.

Ruscello DM, Tekieli ME, Jakomis T et al: The effects of orthognathic surgery on speech production, *Am J Orthod* 89:237-241, 1986.

Ruscello DM, Yancro D, Ghalichebaf M: Cooperative service delivery between a university clinic and school system, *Lang Speech Hear Serv Sch* 26:273-277, 1995.

Shprintzen RJ: *Genetic syndromes and communicative disorders,* San Diego, 1997, Singular.

Shprintzen RJ: *Syndrome identification for speech-language pathology,* San Diego, 2000, Singular.

Shprintzen RJ, Bardach J: *Cleft palate speech management,* St Louis, 1995, Mosby.

Shprintzen RJ, Witzel MA: *Reference guide—delineation and diagnosis of craniofacial syndromes: effect on case management,* Rockville, Md, 1993, American Speech-Language-Hearing Association.

St. Louis KO, Ruscello DM: *Oral speech mechanism screening examination—revised,* Austin, Tex, 2000, Pro-Ed.

Tomes LA, Kuehn DP, Peterson-Falzone SJ: Research considerations for behavioral treatments of velopharyngeal impairment. In Bzoch K, editor: *Communicative disorders related to cleft lip and palate,* ed 5, Austin, Tex, 2004, Pro-Ed.

Trost JE: Articulatory additions to the description of the speech of persons with cleft palate, *Cleft Palate J* 18:193-203, 1981.

Trost-Cardamone JE: The development of speech: assessing cleft palate misarticulations. In Kernahan DA, Rosenstein SW, editors: *Cleft lip and palate,* Baltimore, 1990a, Williams & Wilkins.

Trost-Cardamone JE: Speech: anatomy, physiology, and pathology. In Kernahan DA, Rosenstein SW, editors: *Cleft lip and palate,* Baltimore, 1990b, Williams & Wilkins.

Trost-Cardamone JE: *Speech compensatory misarticulations.* Proceedings of the American Cleft Palate–Craniofacial Association Preconference Symposium, New Orleans, 1997.

Trost-Cardamone JE, Bernthal JE: Articulation assessment procedures and treatment decisions. In Moller KT, Starr CD, editors: *Cleft palate: interdisciplinary issues and treatment,* Austin, Tex, 1993, Pro-Ed.

Vallino LD: Speech, velopharyngeal function, and hearing before and after orthognathic surgery, *J Oral Maxillofac Surg* 48:1274-1281, 1990.

Van Borsel J, Morlion B, Van Snick K et al: Articulation in Beckwith-Wiedemann syndrome, *Am J Speech Lang Pathol* 9:202-213, 2000.

Weng EY, Mortier GR, Graham JM: Beckwith-Wiedemann syndrome, *Clin Pediatr (Phila)* 34: 317-330, 1995.

Williams WN, Waldron CM: Assessment of lingual function when ankyloglossia (tongue-tie) is suspected, *J Am Dent Assoc* 110:353-356, 1985.

Zemlin WR: *Speech and hearing science: anatomy and physiology,* ed 4, Boston, 1998, Allyn & Bacon.

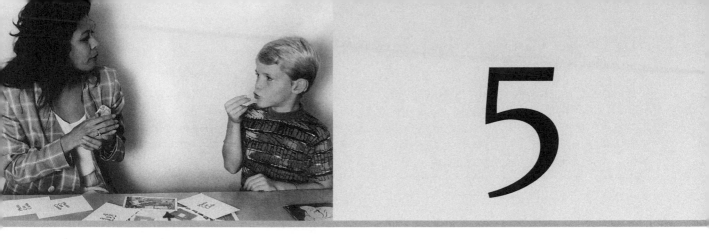

5

Treatment of Children with Hearing Impairment

LEARNING GOALS
- Discuss causes and severity of hearing loss in children.
- Define speech intelligibility, and explain how this index is affected in individuals with hearing loss.

- Describe the relationship between sound system errors and hearing loss.
- Outline the basic treatment of sound system errors, including the

environmental and contextual considerations.
- Discuss the production of both vowels and consonants and ways to teach phonetic and phonemic skills.

Hearing impairment is a variable that can have a definite influence on speech production. A number of investigations have established relationships between hearing impairment and speech production. Findings suggest that a one-to-one relationship does not exist between sound system disorders and the type and severity of hearing loss. Nevertheless, certain treatment variables are important in developing a remediation plan for children with hearing impairment.

Audition is critical to the development of speech and language skills (Northern and Downs, 2002). Children with hearing impairment present a challenge to the practitioner because they have a problem that can have an adverse effect on prespeech and later speech development. Prespeech and speech development proceed in an orderly fashion in normal children; however, the developmental stages of children with hearing impairment are not clearly understood. Research has shown that children with normal hearing discriminate among the different speech sounds across languages before the emergence of their initial word productions (Owens, 2005). When they acquire and develop the phonologies of their linguistic community, they use and discriminate the phonemes that are part of their particular language. Northern and Downs (2002) point out that a great deal of individual learning occurs through the auditory process; consequently, hearing loss can have a significant effect on a child's communication development and overall learning. Before treatment is discussed, the concepts related to treatment are summarized briefly in this chapter to provide a review and develop a foundation for treatment.

Research Note	Research has shown that children with normal hearing discriminate among different speech sounds across languages before their first words emerge.

Owens, 2005.

Table 5-1
Effect of Varying Degrees of Hearing Loss on Speech Perception

AVERAGE HEARING LEVEL (dB)	DEGREE OF HEARING LOSS	CAUSE	EFFECT ON SPEECH PERCEPTION
25-30	Mild hearing loss	Conductive or sensorineural loss	Does not perceive unvoiced sounds and sounds with low intensity
30-50	Moderate hearing loss	Conductive or sensorineural loss	Misses most speech sounds in normal conversation
50-70	Severe hearing loss	Sensorineural or mixed loss	Does not perceive speech sounds in normal conversation
>70	Profound hearing loss	Sensorineural or mixed loss	Does not perceive speech or other sounds

Modified from Northern JL, Downs MP: *Hearing in children,* ed 5, Philadelphia, 2002, Lippincott Williams & Wilkins.

HEARING LOSS

No single cause of hearing loss exists; instead a number of possible causes (e.g., genetic transmission, infections, diseases, trauma) may affect differentially the hearing mechanism (Northern and Downs, 2002). The type and degree of hearing loss have an effect on an individual's ability to perceive and produce speech (Ross et al., 1991). The amount or degree of loss is generally categorized as *mild, moderate, severe,* or *profound.* Children with hearing loss classified in the categories of *mild, moderate,* or *severe* are generally referred to as **hard-of-hearing,** whereas children in the *profound* category are typically described as **deaf.** Table 5-1 was adapted from the work of Northern and Downs (2002) and summarizes the various degrees of hearing loss and their effect on speech perception when early treatment and amplification are not used. As hearing loss increases, the effect on speech perception becomes more severe to the point that the child cannot perceive incoming speech. Hearing loss has a significant effect on the child's production and perception of speech (Bernthal and Bankson, 2004).

The different types of hearing loss may be categorized as *conductive, sensorineural,* or *mixed*. A **conductive hearing loss** is difficulty with sound transmission from the external auditory canal to the inner ear. The inner ear is functioning normally, but some problem adversely affects the air conduction pathway to the cochlea. Roberts and Clarke-Klein (1994) indicate that otitis media is one of the most common childhood illnesses and can have negative effects on hearing. **Otitis media** results in an inflammation of the middle ear and may have no obvious symptoms. Acute otitis media is a condition wherein a sudden inflammation of the middle ear exists, with symptoms of pain, fever, and redness of the tympanic membrane. Otitis media with effusion is present when fluid is found in the middle ear. Many children vacillate between acute otitis media and otitis media with effusion and may not demonstrate frank symptoms such as earache, pulling of the ears, or otorrhea with either middle-ear problem. Hearing loss is generally in the mild to moderate range of impairment, and medical management is necessary.

Research Note   Otitis media, which results in inflammation of the middle ear, is one of the most common childhood illnesses. Children with this illness may exhibit no obvious symptoms.

Roberts and Clarke-Klein, 1994.

Sensorineural hearing loss is the result of damage to the hair cells of the cochlea or the auditory nerve. Sensorineural loss is generally a permanent type of hearing loss that is irreversible (Bess and Humes, 2003). Paterson (1994) states that the management of children with a sensorineural loss in the mild to moderate range includes assistive listening devices, individually tailored educational programs, and speech and language intervention. Children in the severe to profound range also need the same type of assistance, with the addition of intensive language and sound system treatment. A **mixed hearing loss** includes both conductive and sensorineural components, because both contribute to the hearing loss. Management of a mixed hearing loss will depend on the contributions of each component.

Managing children with mild to moderate sensorineural hearing loss includes the use of assistive listening devices, individually tailored educational programs, and speech and language intervention. Those in the severe to profound category need the same type of help, plus intensive language and sound system treatment.

Research **Note**

Paterson, 1994.

SPEECH INTELLIGIBILITY

Speech intelligibility is an index that estimates the speech that can be understood by a listener and is a complex function of intensity, frequency, and time (Flexer, 1994). The person with a hearing loss demonstrates reduced intelligibility because of the reduction of hearing level. Readers should remember that the trends (discussed later in the chapter) are not absolutes; certain sound system disorders do not always correspond to a particular type of loss.

During conversation the average intensity of a person's speech is approximately 65 to 70 dB when about 1 m from the speaker's lips (Flexer, 1994; Northern and Downs, 2002; Tye-Murray, 2004). The **speech intensity (sound pressure)** range from the softest to the loudest speech sound is approximately 46 to 85 dB. Intensity (sound pressure) usually drops about 6 dB with each doubling of distance between the source and receiver. The intensity of individual speech sounds shows approximately a difference of 20 dB between the most intense sounds (vowels) and the least intense sounds (slit fricatives). In order of intensity one finds the following: vowels, diphthongs, sonorants, voiced stops and fricatives, and unvoiced stops and fricatives.

The average intensity of a person's speech is approximately 65 to 70 dB when approximately 1 m from the speaker's lips.

Research **Note**

Flexer, 1994; Northern and Downs, 2002; Tye-Murray, 2004.

If one examines intensity in relation to **frequency,** then one finds that the frequencies below 500 Hz contain 60% of the speech intensity but contribute only 5% to intelligibility (Northern and Downs, 2002). The

Table 5-2
Relationship among Frequency, Speech Intensity, and Speech Intelligibility

FREQUENCY (Hz)	INTENSITY (%)	INTELLIGIBILITY (%)
62-125	5	1
125-250	13	1
250-500	42	3
500-1000	35	35
1000-2000	3	35
2000-4000	1	13
4000-8000	1	12

Data from Northern JL, Downs MP: *Hearing in children,* ed 5, Philadelphia, 2002, Lippincott Williams & Wilkins.

frequencies above 1000 Hz contribute 5% of the speech intensity but account for 60% of the intelligibility as outlined in Table 5-2.

Research Note — Frequencies below 500 Hz contain 60% of the speech intensity but contribute only 5% to speech intelligibility. Furthermore, frequencies above 1000 Hz contribute 5% of speech intensity but account for 60% of intelligibility.

Northern and Downs, 2002.

The sounds of speech contain energy in the frequency range of approximately 100 to 8000 Hz and, as previously mentioned, most of the speech intensity is below 1000 Hz. An individual does not need all frequencies to maintain normal intelligibility because experiments have shown only moderate reductions in intelligibility through the elimination of all frequencies below 1600 Hz or all frequencies above 1600 Hz (Northern and Downs, 2002). Ling (1976) points out that the contribution of individual speech sounds to intelligibility is a very complex consideration because one must understand the interactions of frequency, intensity, and time. In addition, the presence of coarticulation further compounds the already complex problem. Variability is the rule rather than the exception. Consequently, the effects of hearing loss must be examined on an individual basis.

Sound System Errors

Children with hearing loss constitute a heterogeneous group with respect to speech production characteristics, and the speech-language pathologist must be cognizant of such differences (Elfenbein et al., 1994). Tye-Murray (2004) indicated that children with mild to moderate hearing loss constitute a significant population in the schools, and the causes of such loss are thought to reflect middle-ear disease and exposure to noise. One of the most frequent groups to be seen by the practitioner is the group of children with middle-ear disease. Depending on the amount of loss, these children may display fluctuating hearing loss in the mild to moderate range.

Numerous studies have examined potential relationships between otitis media and otitis media with effusion; however, methodological differences, including such factors as study design and subject description, limit the interpretation and generalization of the results (Roberts and Clarke-Klein, 1994; Shriberg et al., 2000). Despite the methodological concerns, reported data suggest that preschool children with recurrent otitis media with effusion are at risk for speech delay (Shriberg et al., 2000). Whether this increased risk is caused by the hearing loss, concomitant illness, allergies, or a combined effect is unclear. In any event, investigators (Roberts and Clarke-Klien, 1994; Tye-Murray, 2004) indicate that sound system disorders for this population consist of fricative and affricate errors, final consonant deletion, cluster reduction, and velar and liquid misarticulations.

Research Note

Data suggest that preschool children with recurrent otitis media with effusion are at risk for speech delay. Sound system disorders, such as fricative and affricate errors, final consonant deletion, cluster reduction, and velar and liquid misarticulations, are found.

Roberts and Clarke-Klein, 1994; Shriberg et al., 2000; Tye-Murray, 2004.

Paterson (1994) summarized the sound system errors found in the speech of children with severe to profound hearing loss. Typical patterns of **segmental errors** include both vowel and consonant involvement. Vowel errors include substitutions that may differ in terms of tense versus lax with adjacent vowels, neutralization to schwa-like approximations, substitutions that differ significantly in terms of placement (i.e., front and back), vowel-diphthong substitutions, distortions of intended vowels, and omission of vowels. In addition, some investigators have reported that hypernasal resonance accompanies vowel production. In most cases the resonance problem is a lack of velopharyngeal control because of presenting hearing loss, not a velopharyngeal valving problem, which would require surgical or prosthetic correction (Ling, 1976). Consonant misarticulations consist of substitution confusions such as voiced and voiceless, nasal and oral, fricative and stop, the deletion of prevocalic and postvocalic consonants, and distortions such as hypernasality and nasal emission. Table 5-3 outlines sound system errors in relation to children's hearing loss from mild to profound.

In addition to segmental errors, children with severe to profound hearing loss exhibit problems with suprasegmental features or prosody (Ling, 1976). **Prosodic features** are superimposed on words, phrases, and sentences and provide the flow or organization of speech production. Prosodic features include pitch, loudness, stress, duration, and vocal quality. Investigators (Paterson, 1994) have identified a variety of problems in this population such as inappropriate breath control, incorrect use of pause, vocal errors including lack of pitch variation and quality (i.e., breathiness, harshness), problems with the duration of stressed and unstressed syllables, and rate of syllable production.

Treatment of Sound System Errors

A treatment program for children with hearing impairment must encompass those variables that will facilitate the acquisition of correct speech (Ling, 2002). Implementation of a program should incorporate environmental, contextual, and therapeutic variables. Environmental variables pertain to the therapy and classroom conditions for the hearing-impaired child. Contextual and therapeutic variables are treatment based and deal with the structuring of target stimuli to maximize residual hearing and the actual content being taught. The speech-language pathologist needs to work closely with the child's educational audiologist, classroom teacher, and caregivers in the process of communication intervention.

Table 5-3
Summary of Sound System Errors as a Function of Degree of Hearing Loss

AVERAGE HEARING LEVEL (dB)	DEGREE OF LOSS	CAUSE	SOUND SYSTEM ERRORS
25-30	Mild hearing loss	Conductive or sensorineural loss	Fricatives, affricates, final consonant deletion, clusters, and /r/, /l/ errors
30-50	Moderate hearing loss	Conductive or sensorineural loss	Same as previous errors
50-70	Severe hearing loss	Sensorineural or mixed loss	Vowel substitutions, distortions, omissions, and hypernasality; consonant substitutions, distortions, omissions, and nasal emission; errors of prosody
>70	Profound hearing loss	Sensorineural or mixed loss	Same as previous errors

Data from Paterson MM: Articulation and phonological disorders in hearing-impaired school-aged children with severe and profound sensorineural losses. In Bernthal J, Bankson N, editors: *Child phonology: characteristics, assessment, and intervention with special populations,* New York, 1994, Thieme Medical.

Environmental Considerations. The practitioner must maximize the treatment conditions (Box 5-1). Flexer (1994) indicates that listening skills for a hearing-impaired child need to be optimized. That is, the clinician must ensure that the child is receiving appropriate amplification, that any ear-related medical problems are being managed, and that

> **BOX 5-1** *Environmental Treatment Considerations for the Child with Hearing Impairment*
>
> **Pretreatment Considerations**
> - Child is receiving appropriate amplification.
> - Ear-related medical problems are followed.
> - Home and school are controlled to minimize extraneous noise.
>
> **Treatment Considerations**
> - Clinician should ensure his or her face is visible to the child.
> - Clinician should speak at a moderate rate.
> - Clinician should use a slight pause at the informational boundaries of utterances.
> - Clinician should obtain the attention of the child before speaking.

the child's learning contexts are controlled for extraneous noise. Central to treatment is conducting therapy in a quiet environment with the client's assistive listening device operating appropriately. Ling and Ling (1978) recommend that the practitioner conduct the Five Sound Test before each treatment session (see Additional Teaching Activities, later in this chapter). The intensity level of the practice should be about 30 dB above the ambient noise level. This is important because the range of intensity across speech sounds is approximately 20 dB. If the ambient noise level in the room is 50 dB, then the loudest sounds must approach 70 dB for the faintest sounds to be above the ambient noise level.

When working with the child, the clinician should ensure his or her face is visible and that no visual distractions, such as chewing gum (Tye-Murray, 2004), occur. Hands are kept away from the face, and the clinician uses a moderate rate of speech so that visual production cues are available to the client. Speaking rates that are either too fast or too slow can be confusing. Pausing should occur at phrase and sentence boundaries to allow the individual sufficient processing time. In normal speaking, one pauses at grammatical boundaries; the clinician should incorporate this into his or her treatment with the client. Finally, one should gain the child's attention before speaking to him or her. The clinician should also request feedback from the client regarding variables such as speech rate, intensity, and message clarification, as well as discover whether the child is having problems understanding anything before initiating treatment on that day.

BOX 5-2   *Effect of Hearing Loss on the Speech Perception of the Child with Hearing Impairment*

Contextual Considerations

Profound Hearing Loss
- Frequency and intensity information is very limited.
- Some durational information can be perceived.

Severe Hearing Loss
- Spectral information for the perception of consonant manner of production may be available for most sound classes.
- Discrimination of place of articulation for different consonant manner may be difficult.

Moderate Hearing Loss
- Manner of consonant production and voicing cues can be perceived.
- Perception of place of articulation may be a problem, particularly for stops and fricatives.

Contextual Considerations. The practitioner must be cognizant of the acoustic features of the speech signal to use the client's residual hearing (DeFilipo and Clark, 1993). Revoile (1999) points out that persons with hearing impairment have limitations in the perception of important speech intensity and frequency information. When providing treatment services, the practitioner must be aware of the limitations and develop treatment stimuli that maximize available acoustic information. That is, the practitioner must use the client's residual hearing (Ling, 2002). Box 5-2 summarizes the contextual considerations.

Although each client is different, Revoile (1999) presents some hypothetical data that aid in understanding the effect of hearing loss on speech perception. Individuals with profound hearing loss in the range of approximately 90- to 115-dB hearing level are limited in their perception of acoustic information. They typically cannot discriminate among speech sounds without the benefit of visual cues and must use **amplification** as an adjunct to lip-reading (De Fillipo and Clark, 1993). **Spectral information** is very limited, but some **durational information** may be available for these clients. This means that manner of sound production and voicing cues will be difficult to perceive even with amplification. Some clients may be able to discriminate postvocalic stops and fricatives based on vowel duration (i.e., vowels are longer in duration when they precede voiced rather voiceless consonants). Voicing differences for stops in the prevocalic and intervocalic positions may also be differentiated on the basis of **voice onset time (VOT).** When articulating **plosives,** durational differences exist in the stop burst and start of the vowel articulation, which differ depending on whether the plosive is voiced or voiceless. Voiceless plosives have a longer duration between the onset of the burst and the initiation of voicing for the vowel sound.

Research Note	Individuals with profound hearing loss in the range of approximately 90- to 115-dB hearing loss are limited in their perception of acoustic information. They typically cannot discriminate among speech sounds without the benefit of visual cues and often need amplification to accompany lip-reading.

De Fillipo and Clark, 1993; Revoile, 1999.

Clients with severe hearing loss in the range of 65- to 90-dB hearing level can vary significantly in terms of speech perception because of a number of factors including variability in dynamic range (Revoile, 1999). **Dynamic range** is the difference in intensity between a person's threshold of sensitivity for sound and the level at which the intensity of the sound becomes uncomfortable (Tye-Murray, 2004). A limited dynamic range would restrict the degree of amplification that could be used. Low-frequency information is likely available and will enable the perception of some glides and nasals and voicing cues. The availability of low-frequency information may also enable discrimination of glides versus stop and fricative categories. Within the different manner categories, place of articulation may be problematic.

Research Note	Individuals with severe hearing loss in the range of 65- to 90-dB hearing level vary significantly in speech perception skills, due in part to restrictions in dynamic range—the difference in intensity between a person's threshold of sensitivity for sound and the level at which the intensity becomes uncomfortable.

Revoile, 1999; Tye-Murray, 2004.

Revoile (1999) indicates that clients in the moderate range of hearing loss (45- to 65-dB hearing level) typically do not have dynamic range problems that adversely affect amplification. In many cases, amplified speech may approach normal hearing levels, provided the loss is a flat configuration. A sloping hearing configuration with increasing loss at the higher frequencies may prevent the perception of high-frequency information and thus reduce the number of acoustic cues that are available to the hearing-impaired listener. Generally, manner and voicing cues are available to the moderately impaired listener, but place of articulation may be problematic (particularly for fricatives and plosives).

Hearing loss has a negative effect on speech perception, and practitioners need to be aware of such limitations so that they may structure teaching content appropriately. Ling (1976, 2002) has carefully considered contextual factors and formulated a series of guidelines that can be used for treatment. However, reviewing the acoustics of vowel and consonant production is necessary to provide the reader with a context for using the client's residual hearing in teaching speech sound production skills.

Vowel and Consonant Production

Vowels and diphthongs are voiced sounds produced by selectively amplifying the complex aperiodic sound source (laryngeal tone) through cavity resonance (Ling, 1976). The vocal tract assumes a certain configuration primarily as a result of movements of the lips and tongue; the result is the creation of **formants,** or bands of sound energy at certain frequency regions. Listeners identify the different vowels and diphthongs through auditory perception of the formants. Listeners can generally differentiate among vowels, if they can perceive the first and second vowel formants. In addition, vowels also exhibit **vocalic transitions,** which are alterations in vowel formant energy. The acoustic changes are the physiologic result of vowel movement to or away from an adjacent consonant articulation. Vocalic transitions provide listeners with important cues in the perception of neighboring consonant sounds. Vowels are classified according to the point of constriction of the tongue in the vocal tract (front, central, back), degree of constriction or tongue height (high, middle, low), and presence or absence of lip rounding. Diphthongs are produced by moving or gliding from one vowel target to another. It must be noted that a great deal of variability exists among English speakers with respect to vowel production, and dialect variation is also often reflected in vowel production differences.

The front vowels are /i, I, e, ɛ, æ/, and they differ according to tongue height (Shriberg and Kent, 1995). In addition, the lips are slightly spread when articulating the sounds. If a speaker produces the vowels in isolation starting with /i/ and moves the front part of the tongue, then he or she will feel the tongue moving downward in addition to slight jaw opening. He or she will also perceive differences in tongue tension when producing the different front vowels. The vowel pairs /i, I/ and /e, ɛ/ are articulated at a relatively similar point of articulation, but muscular tension of the tongue is present during the production of /i/ and /e/. The muscular tension results in a production that has more intensity and is longer in duration than its lax counterpart. Acoustically, the first formant of front vowels is less than 1000 Hz, but the second formant is generally above 1000 Hz for the various front vowels. This is an important consideration in the structuring of stimuli when a client has little residual hearing above 1000 Hz.

Shriberg and Kent (1995) indicate that constriction at the dorsum area of the tongue results in the production of **back vowels.** Another important production feature of back vowels is that they are produced with lip rounding. The production feature of lip rounding acts to lengthen the vocal tract, and the acoustic result is a lowering of the first and second formants. The back vowels in order of high to low tongue height are /u, ʊ, o, ɔ, ɑ/. The degree of lip rounding decreases with lowering of the tongue. The vowel pairs /u, ʊ/ are **tense/lax pairs.** The first formant frequency values are below 1000 Hz, and the second formant values are near or slightly above 1000 Hz. The acoustic properties of back vowels are facilitative for clients with little residual hearing above 1000 Hz.

Research Note	Back vowels are produced via placement of the tongue dorsum. Lip rounding, which acts to lengthen the vocal tract, is also a feature of back vowels.

Shriberg and Kent, 1995.

The central vowels /ə, ʌ, ɚ, ɝ/ are produced with the tongue positioned approximately in the center of the oral cavity. Shriberg and Kent (1995) indicate that tongue height does not vary significantly among these vowels; the vowel /ʌ/ is typically produced with a tongue position that is lower and farther back than the other central vowels. The r-colored vowels /ɝ, ɚ/ are tense/lax pairs. Stress or prominence plays a role in the perception of the different central vowels. The vowels /ʌ, ɝ/ are used in stressed syllables, whereas the vowels /ə, ɚ/ are used in syllables that do not receive primary stress. The word *ruckus* /ˈrʌk əs/ is an example of the two central vowels /ʌ, ə/ in context and contrasts the stressed syllable from the unstressed. Formant values for

---

> **BOX 5-3**   *Consonants versus Vowels*
>
> Consonants differ from vowels in the following three ways:
> 1. Physiologically, they are made with complete or partial occlusion of the vowel tract.
> 2. Acoustically, they show significant variation in intensity from sound to sound.
> 3. They exhibit significant variation in duration and frequency characteristics.

---

central vowels are similar to those of the front vowels. The first formant is below 1000 Hz, whereas second formant is above 1000 Hz.

Gliding from one vowel position to another produces **diphthongs.** A slow gliding movement or vocalic transition from one vowel point (onglide) to another vowel point (offglide) occurs. The tongue elevates when moving from the onglide to the offglide position for English diphthongs. The diphthongs include /aɪ, aʊ/ and /ɔɪ/.

Consonants differ from vowels in a number of ways (Box 5-3). Physiologically, they are made with complete or partial occlusion of the vocal tract (Kent, 1997). Acoustically, they show significant variation in intensity from sound to sound, and they also exhibit significant variation in duration and frequency characteristics. These differences present challenges to the practitioner when treating the hearing-impaired child. For the purposes of this chapter, consonants are discussed in relation to the production features of manner, place, and voicing. If one conceptualizes consonant sounds on a continuum of closed-open constriction of the vocal tract, then the order is stops, affricates, fricatives, nasals, and semivowels.

Stop sounds are produced with a complete occlusion of the vocal tract. An occlusion exists that is held or maintained, the release of which creates a noise burst (Borden et al., 2006). The stops (according to place of articulation) consist of the bilabials /p, b/, lingua-alveolars /t, d/, and the linguavelars /k, g/. A glottal stop /ʔ/ also exists in English but is nonphonemic; in some cases this stop is used to initiate vowels at the beginning of words and may also be used as an allophone of /t, d/ in some dialects of English. The glottal stop is produced by occluding the airstream at the level of glottis and then releasing the energy. Glottal stops are voiceless sounds. Acoustically, a silent period occurs that marks the occlusion of vocal tract for stops. However, voiced stops /b, d, g/ will show voicing (fundamental frequency) during a portion of or across the entire silent period. At the time of stop release, a noise burst occurs that is very transient and may encompass a wide range of frequencies with differences in intensity. The noise burst for bilabial stops is approximately 500 to 1500 Hz, whereas the burst for the lingua-alveolars is generally above 4000 Hz, with an additional concentration of energy near 500 Hz. The linguavelar stops show variation because the noise burst is influenced by the second formant frequencies of the following vowel, but noise burst energy is generally present from 1500 to 4000 Hz.

Research Note	Stop sounds are produced with complete occlusion of the vocal tract. The occlusion is held or maintained before being released, creating a noise burst.

Borden et al., 2006.

The **affricates** /tʃ, dʒ/ are produced with a complete occlusion (such as a stop) and a gradual release (as in the case of a fricative). Borden and colleagues (2006) indicate that a complete occlusion of the vocal tract occurs near the posterior alveolar region and then a gradual release of the tongue back toward the hard palate. The acoustic features of affricates show a noise burst with the release and then the fricative noise period that corresponds to the gradual release. Hearing up to and above 1000 Hz is necessary for the perception of affricates.

Research Note	In the production of English affricates, the vocal tract is completely occluded near the posterior alveolar region, followed by a gradual release of the tongue back toward the hard palate.

Borden et al., 2006.

Forcing the airstream through narrow constrictions within the vocal tract produces the aperiodic sound generation characteristic of fricatives (Borden et al., 2006). The voiced or voiceless breathstream creates a turbulent noise or frication. In English, the points of constriction for the fricatives include labiodental, linguadental, alveolar, palatal, and glottal. The sounds corresponding to the points of articulation are /f, v, θ, ð, s, z, ʃ, ʒ, h/. Acoustically, the /f, v, θ, ð/ are referred to as **slit fricatives** because the constriction for the sounds is more elliptical than round in shape. The configuration is not conducive to the generation of a turbulent noise source, and no resonating cavity exists anterior to the points of articulation. The result is very low spectral energy or intensity spread across a wide band of frequencies that ranges from 1500 to 7500 Hz. The **interdental fricatives** are similar, with low spectral energy starting around 1000 Hz and extending upward. The **alveolar fricatives** and **palatal fricatives** are made with a more circular orifice, and a resonating cavity exists anterior to the points of articulation. A majority of the sound energy for the alveolars is above 3000 Hz, whereas the major concentration of sound energy for the palatals is around 2000 Hz. The glottal /h/ is produced by forcing the breathstream through the approximated vocal folds. Generally the vocal tract assumes the shape of the vowel that follows production of the /h/ when /h/ is articulated. Although sound energy is spread throughout the spectra, concentrations exist near 1000 and 1700 Hz during /h/ articulation.

The nasal sounds /m, n, ŋ/ are voiced sounds and the only sounds in English produced with nasal resonance (Shriberg and Kent, 1995). An occlusion of the oral cavity and communication with the nasal cavity exists. The oral cavity occlusion may be at the lips /m/, the alveolar ridge /n/, or the velum /ŋ/. Physiologically, the unique production characteristics result in pharyngeal, oral cul-de-sac, and nasal resonation. The acoustic products are the presence of nasal murmur, damping, and antiresonances. **Nasal murmur** is the presence of a major low-frequency resonance or nasal formant. In addition, all formants are dampened or reduced in overall energy and have wide bandwidths because of the dampening. Finally, **antiresonances,** which are regions in the frequency spectra severely attenuated by nasal resonation, are present in the spectra of nasal consonants. Nasals generally exhibit enhanced energy below 3000 Hz, an antiresonance region near 500 Hz, and a reduction in interformant fill between 1000 Hz and 2500 Hz.

The nasal sounds /m, n, ŋ/ are voiced and are the only sounds in the English language that are produced with nasal resonance.

Research Note

Shriberg and Kent, 1995.

Borden and colleagues (2006) indicate that the semivowels are labeled as such because their formant structure is very similar to vowels and diphthongs. The **semivowels** /w, j, l, r/ (similar to the other consonants) release and arrest syllables; they do not function as syllable nuclei.

Many sources on speech production identify /w, j/ as **glides** and /r, l/ as **liquids.** A characteristic feature of the sounds is a brief steady-state point of articulation and slow movement to and away from the steady state. The /w/ is produced with lip rounding and linguapalatal movement; the vocal tract approximation is similar to the vowel /u/. The /j/ sound is classified as a *palatal glide* and has a vocal tract configuration similar to /i/. The first formant values for both /w, j/ are low, with the brief steady state at approximately 250 to 300 Hz. The second formant values differ, with the /w/ value starting at around 600 Hz and the /j/ value at approximately 2300 Hz.

Research Note	The semivowel is so named because its formant structure is very similar to both vowels and diphthongs.

Borden et al., 2006.

The liquids /r, l/ demonstrate variable placement that depends on their position within the syllable. In the prevocalic position, /r/ is often produced with a grooved tongue tip that approximates but does not come in contact with the alveolar ridge. Some speakers produce the /r/ in a retroflexed position in which tongue tip curling exists and a more posterior point of production is found. In the postvocalic position, /r/ is frequently produced with elevation of the tongue dorsum. The tongue tip contacts the alveolar ridge in production of the /l/, and raising of the tongue dorsum occurs when articulated in the postvocalic position of syllables. The first and second formant values for /r, l/ are similar. The first is near or above 350 Hz, whereas the second is near or above 950 Hz. The third formant is an important feature in discriminating the two sounds from each other. Formant 3 for /r/ begins at about 1500 Hz and then moves to the third formant of the adjacent vowel. The /l/ shows a short steady state at approximately 3000 Hz.

Figure 5-1 provides a broad overview of the oral cavity and the points of articulation.

Teaching Vowels

In many cases the teaching of speech sound production skills to individuals with hearing impairment requires the incorporation of both phonetic and phonological teaching components. As Ling (2002) points out, correct phonetic placement must be taught if the sound is absent

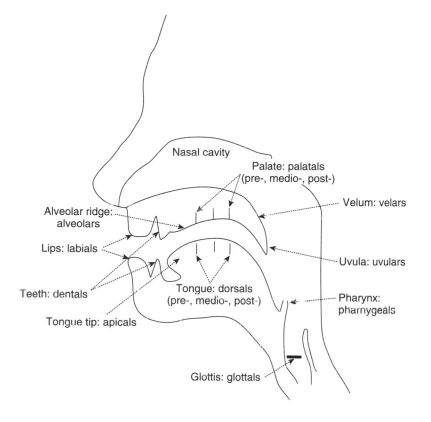

Figure 5-1 ▪ Structures of the oral cavity and places of articulation. (Redrawn from Bauman-Waengler J: *Articulatory and phonological impairments: a clinical focus,* ed 2, Boston, 2004, Allyn & Bacon.)

from the child's inventory, but then the sound must be used in the appropriate context so that the speaker develops the phonemic contrast. The hearing impairment places constraints on both phonetic and phonemic learning for the child. Consequently, treatment must use content that exploits the child's residual hearing through context considerations. It should also be noted that children with hearing impairment—particularly those with a profound degree of loss—frequently require treatment for both vowels and consonants, and the practitioner should refer to the acoustics and physiology of normal speech sound production discussed previously.

| Research Note | Correct phonetic placement must be taught if a sound is absent from the child's inventory. The sound also must be used in the appropriate context to ensure that the speaker develops the phonemic contrast. |

Ling, 2002.

Teaching the placement and correct use of vowels is a requisite goal for many profoundly hearing-impaired children. Ling (2002) indicates that the most important variable in vowel production is the point of maximum constriction of the tongue. To achieve correct placement of the tongue in coordination with the lips and jaw, Ling recommends that the client be taught a resting placement that will facilitate different vowel placements. According to the author, the client must be taught to place the tongue tip in contact with or in close proximity to the lower incisors as a resting placement. The jaw is slightly open to expose the lower teeth and tongue. In this position the client can move the tongue and lips to a point that corresponds to the appropriate placement for a particular vowel. Exaggerated movements of the jaw are avoided when teaching the placement of specific vowels because such exaggeration could cause vowel distortion. Ling also recommends that vowels be introduced in sets that include vowels and diphthongs. The sets vary in terms of vowel production parameters discussed so that point of constriction (front-central-back), degree of constriction (high-mid-low), and lip rounding are considered in creating the different practice sets. The vowel teaching sets, in order, are /ɑ, I, u/, /ɔ, ɛ, ʊ, ɪ/, /æ, ʌ, o, e/, and /ɝ, ə, ɚ/.

| Research Note | Exaggerated movements of the lips, jaw, or tongue must be avoided when teaching vowel placements. |

Ling, 2002.

The reader should remember that correct vowel placement facilitates intelligibility and also provides important acoustic information for the perception of the intended vowel and adjacent consonant speech sounds. If the client has residual hearing up to the range of 3000 Hz, then the first two vowel formants for all vowels are within the range of audibility; therefore imitation can be used with phonetic placement cues to achieve correct vowel production. The use of whisper is also a strategy that the practitioner may want to consider because harmonic structure

---

BOX 5-4 *Four Steps to Phonetic Teaching for Vowels*

1. Use auditory stimulation to elicit a vowel sound in isolation.
   - Use phonetic placement techniques if necessary.
   - Use tactile stimulation if necessary.
2. Perform sustained practice with the vowel in isolation.
3. Practice in the context of CV contexts.
4. Instruct the client to use the acquired vowels in words, using contrast with nonadjacent vowels /bit-but/.

Data from Ling D: *Speech and the hearing-impaired child: theory and practice,* Washington, DC, 1976, The Alexander Graham Bell Association for the Deaf and Hard of Hearing.

is eliminated and the second formant may be more prominent to the client (Ling, 1976). The use of whisper may also facilitate diphthong production because acoustic information regarding movement from one vowel to another may become more salient for the client. If the range of audibility is reduced, then vowel confusions will occur because F2 information cannot be perceived and some vowels share similar first formant frequencies. The reader should keep in mind that, as an aggregate, back vowels have a lower F2 than front vowels and can serve as the initial context for teaching production skills.

When residual hearing is limited, it may be necessary to use other teaching techniques to achieve correct vowel production. For example, the practitioner may want to produce a specific vowel while having the child touch the tongue to develop the percept of the production. Following the illustration, the child can be instructed to touch his or her tongue and attempt production. Other teaching techniques (e.g., models of the articulators, diagrams) may also be used to explain and illustrate correct placement for a specific vowel.

Ling (1976) recommends that phonetic teaching for individual vowels be carried out in four steps (Box 5-4). First, he recommends the use of auditory stimulation to elicit a vowel sound in isolation. If auditory stimulation is not successful, then phonetic placement techniques may be used to achieve correct production in isolation. Tactile stimulation such as using the fingers to position the articulators or using visual signals to cue a particular vowel may also be used. Perigoe (2002) recommends that if tactile or visual cues (or both) are used, they should be faded as soon as possible.

When the client is capable of producing the vowel in isolation, the second step consists of sustained practice with the vowel in isolation.

Practice consists of producing vowels and sustaining them for approximately 3 seconds. The reader should note that diphthongs cannot be prolonged in the same manner because movement occurs from one vowel point of articulation to another. The vowels are to be sustained in isolation practice; however, the practitioner must critically monitor the productions to avoid movement from the point of constriction and the production of a diphthong.

The third step of the practice paradigm is practice in the context of CV contexts. The bilabial /b/ is used initially because it provides visual cues for the client. After production is achieved with the bilabial, other consonant sounds may be introduced and practiced.

The fourth step is phonemic based and requires the client to use the acquired vowels in words using contrast with nonadjacent vowels /bit-but/. Pictures are used in minimal pair contrast so that the child is confronted with the phonemic differences (Abraham, 1993; Gibbons and Beck, 2002; Robbins, 2000). The initial teaching steps are phonetic based, and the final step in the treatment is phonemic based. The rationale is to teach the necessary phonetic placement skills and then develop the appropriate phonemic contrasts. After the development of vowel contrast, activities are introduced for the purpose of transfer to communicative situations (Perigoe, 2002). Actual situations, role-playing, and the client's interests can be used as topics for transfer to communicative situations. Clinician feedback of the child's productions is very important in the achievement of vowel targets during the stages of vowel teaching; however, the child should also engage in self-evaluation of their practice productions during treatment (Paterson, 1994).

Because the clients are hearing impaired, the practitioner should have the client vary the duration of the vowels and encourage the client to produce the vowels with variations in vocal pitch (Paterson, 1994). This is an important feature because many hearing-impaired clients exhibit problems in using various suprasegmental features in their speech. Automatic activities such as reciting poems and rhymes can be used to practice the production of different sounds in contexts that emphasize the suprasegmental aspects of vowel production (Ertmer et al., 2002). The clinician must also monitor productions for hypernasality. Oftentimes, functional hypernasality is present in the vowel productions of clients with hearing impairment. In such a case, the client needs instruction to produce vowels without hypernasality.

| Research Note | The clinician should instruct clients to vary the duration of vowels and encourage them to produce vowels with variations in vocal pitch. |

Paterson, 1994.

> **BOX 5-5** *Summary of Vowel Teaching Paradigm*
>
> **Teaching Steps**
> 1. Teach tongue-resting placement.
> 2. Introduce different vowel teaching subsets, and conduct phonetic practice.
>   a. Practice isolation.
>   b. Practice sustained isolation.
>   c. Practice in context of CV syllables.
> 3. Introduce phonemic practice with the target vowel in contrast with other vowels.
> 4. Incorporate practice activities to facilitate target use in spontaneous speech.
> 5. Introduce pitch variation in phonetic and phonemic teaching.
> 6. Modify teaching as a function of different vowel production errors.

In summary, the client initially is taught correct placement skills; he or she then practices sustained vowels in isolation, produces the vowels in words starting with bilabials, and finally practices the vowels in word contrast with nonadjacent vowels (Box 5-5).

The reader should note that the previously discussed vowel teaching methods may need to be modified for clients with other vowel problems, such as those discussed earlier in Sound System Errors or identified by other authors (Paterson, 1994).

Teaching Consonants

Consonants differ significantly from vowels in terms of production characteristics and resulting acoustic output. As discussed, consonants are produced via differing constrictions of the vocal tract; some are produced with voicing, whereas others are not. Moreover, adjacent acoustic vowel information is very important in the perception of different consonants (Borden et al., 2006). In this chapter, the discussion of consonant teaching deals with the production features of manner, place, and voicing, as well as the perceptual information available to the speaker across the spectra.

Ling (2002) has indicated that manner cues are the most important cues in the perception of words in the English language, and a great deal of acoustic information regarding manner is available in the low-frequency range of 1000 Hz and below. Different consonant classes exhibit invariant cues that are distinctive to a sound class and help in the discrimination of that particular sound class. For example, an invariant cue of fricative manner is the creation of a turbulent noise source, which is produced by forcing sound energy through a narrow constriction. Consonants also show variant cues, which differ as a function of coarticulatory influences. An example is the fact that vowels occurring before fricatives are generally longer in duration and intensity than those preceding stops. Information regarding place of articulation is generally available via vocalic transitions, particularly in the second and third formant transitions. Consequently, acoustic information in the middle frequencies to high frequencies is requisite to place perception of consonants. Voicing information is provided by low-frequency acoustic energy, and such information is generally available to clients with residual hearing in the lower frequency range.

Research Note	Manner of production cues are believed to be the most important cues in the perception of words in the English language, and much acoustic information regarding manner is available in the low-frequency range of 1000 Hz and below.

Ling, 2002.

According to the work of Ling (1976, 2002), consonants should be introduced in groups that include different manner of production. The more visual sounds such as the bilabials /p, b, m, w/, labiodentals /f, v/, linguadentals /θ, ð/, and the glottal /h/ are taught initially and then followed by the alveolars /s, z, t, d, n, l/ and palatals /j, ʃ, ʒ/. The final set contains the alveolar /r/, palatals /tʃ, dʒ/, and the velars /k, g, ŋ/. The teaching of consonants follows steps similar to those described in the vowel-teaching discussion. The sound is first taught in isolation (if a continuant) or in the context of a syllable (if not a continuant). Auditory stimulation is used initially as the method for sound elicitation. As recommended with vowel teaching, whispered speech stimuli may be more salient to the client because it acts to accentuate formant frequencies. If the client cannot produce the target via auditory stimulation, then other techniques are used. Auditory stimulation may be followed by phonetic placement techniques. If unsuccessful, then tactile stimulation techniques such as using the fingers to position the articulators or identifying the breathstream characteristics of a sound can be used. The reader should note that some authors such as Perigoe (2002) recommend against practitioners placing their fingers in the client's mouth. Visual signals to cue a particular consonant may also be used. As mentioned with vowels, if tactile or visual cues (or both) are used, then they must be faded as soon as possible.

Some clinicians do not recommend the placement of fingers in a client's mouth as a tactile stimulation technique.	*Research* Note

Perigoe, 1992.

After the successful acquisition of the sound in isolation or in a syllable if not a continuant, practice is designed for transfer to different phonetic contexts with appropriate prosodic variations. The client first practices the target in the prevocalic position in the context of the vowels /i, u, ɑ/. However, Perigoe (2002) recommends that fricatives, nasals, and liquids be taught initially in the postvocalic position.

This is followed by repetitive strings of syllables /bi, bi, bi/ and then repetitive strings with consonant and differing vowel combinations /bi, bu, be, bo/. The final step in this sequence is the production of syllable repetitions in the context of different vowels with variation in inflection. The clinician should provide clear and concise feedback to the client, who should judge his or her own productions for accuracy.

After the client has achieved phonetic production of a particular target, activities are conducted to build phonemic skill or phonological reorganization of the ambient language. As discussed with vowel teaching, the clinician must introduce contrast so that the acoustic and meaning contrasts are presented to the client. For example, a client may confuse /ʃ/ for /tʃ/, so minimal pairs may be used to contrast the manner substitution with the desired target. Minimal pairs may also be used to stabilize other errors such as the voiced versus voiceless contrast and place contrasts within or among manner of production categories. Additional activities such as incorporation of the targets in spontaneous activities such as conversation, narration, and topic description can be used to establish correct phonemic production. A summary of the teaching steps is presented in Box 5-6.

Additional Teaching Activities

In addition to the specific activities discussed for vowel and consonant teaching, the following general principles apply to the treatment of clients with hearing impairment (Chin, 2002; Paterson, 1994; Perigoe, 2002):

BOX 5-6   *Teaching Considerations for Consonants*

Phonetic
1. Introduce visible consonants followed by consonants that are not highly visible in different designated subsets.
2. Teach the sound in isolation if necessary.
   a. Use auditory stimulation.
   b. If auditory stimulation is not successful, then use teaching techniques in the listed hierarchy.
3. Conduct initial phonetic practice in syllables with the vowels /i, u, ɑ/.
4. Continue to practice with the target sound in repetitive strings with the same vowel.
5. Shift practice to the target in repetitive strings with different vowels.
6. Practice with the target and different vowels, with the emphasis on prosodic variation.

Phonemic
1. Use minimal pair contrast.
2. Use spontaneous activities such as conversation to establish correct phonemic production and suprasegmental variation.

- Before beginning each treatment session, check the client's auditory reception via his or her assistive listening device using the Five Sound Test (Ling & Ling, 1978). The sounds /u, ɑ, i, s, ʃ/ are produced for the client to repeat. Visual cues may be provided; however, presentation of cues must be consistent across sessions. The stimuli represent a wide range in the speech frequencies, thus providing a screening of auditory reception. Changes in the screening test indicate the need for evaluating the assistive listening device and audiological testing.
- The clinician should be positioned beside the client (not in front) when working with him or her. If visual cues are necessary, the clinician can turn toward the client and furnish the appropriate visual information. Speech movements should never be exaggerated, and appropriate speech models must be provided.
- Provide the client with immediate feedback regarding performance. Positive cues such as "good job" and "that's very good" should follow correct performance. Identify errors and provide appropriate feedback to the client.

- Conduct periodic probes of the client's performance so that adjustments can be made in the treatment program.
- Conduct treatment sessions for short periods of time, rather than extended periods. In addition, spread short treatment sessions throughout an instructional day whenever possible.
- Target sessions toward multiple goals rather than working on a single goal. For example, one goal might involve phonetic practice with one target, phonemic contrast with another set of targets, and conversational practice with different targets.
- Try to identify, through phonetic transcription, the different errors used by the client. These data can provide important information regarding the use of phonetic teaching (correct sound placement), phonemic teaching (phonological reorganization), or both.
- Involve the classroom teacher in the treatment process, and take the treatment to the classroom.
- Involve the client's parents in the treatment process so that they may reinforce what is being covered in treatment. In addition, ensure that appropriate instruction is provided to the parents to ensure consistency between the school and home.

SUMMARY

Teaching speech skills to clients with hearing impairment is only one aspect of communication instruction for this population; however, this component of treatment is very important to the overall language and literacy process. This chapter provides information that the speech-language pathologist may use in the treatment of sound system disorders with children who are hearing impaired. Carney and Moeller (1998) conducted an extensive review of educational, language, and speech treatment investigations for children with hearing loss. The authors concluded that hearing impairment in the mild to profound range of loss has an adverse effect on a child's hearing, speech and language, educational achievement, and social-emotional growth. The authors further stated that a number of interventions are available, including sensory aids, different communication modalities, and various academic curricula; however, to date no definitive research supports one particular treatment over another. Hearing loss is a sensory variable that challenges the skills and knowledge of the speech-language pathologist. The treatment recommendations included in this chapter are based on using the child's residual hearing, treatment stimuli that exploit residual hearing, and teaching techniques that facilitate phonetic and phonemic learning.

Research Note	In an extensive review of educational, language, and speech treatment for children with hearing loss, researchers concluded that hearing impairment in the mild to profound range of loss has an adverse effect on a child's hearing, speech, language, educational achievement, and social-emotional growth.

Carney and Moeller, 1998.

REFERENCES

Abraham S: Differential treatment of phonological disability in children with impaired hearing who were trained orally, *Am J Speech Lang Pathol* 2:23-30, 1993.

Bernthal JE, Bankson NW: *Articulation and phonological disorders,* ed 5, Boston, 2004, Allyn & Bacon.

Bess FH, Humes LE: *Audiology: the fundamentals,* ed 3, Philadelphia, 2003, Lippincott Williams & Wilkins.

Borden GJ, Harris KS, Raphael LJ: *Speech science primer: physiology, acoustics, & perception,* ed 5, Baltimore, 2006, Williams & Wilkins.

Carney AE, Moeller MP: Treatment efficacy: hearing loss in children, *J Speech Lang Hear Res* 41:561-584, 1998.

Chin SB: Aspects of stop consonant production by pediatric users of cochlear implants, *Lang Speech Hear Serv Sch* 33:38-51, 2002.

DeFillipo C, Clark C: Use of ambiguous visual stimuli to demonstrate the value of acoustic cues in speech perception, *J Commun Disord* 26:29-51, 1993.

Elfenbein JL, Hardin-Jones MA, Davis JM: Oral communication skills of children who are hard of hearing, *J Speech Hear Res* 37:216-226, 1994.

Ertmer DJ, Leonard JS, Pachuilo ML: Communication intervention for children with cochlear implants: two case studies, *Lang Speech Hear Serv Sch* 33:205-217, 2002.

Flexer C: *Facilitating hearing and listening in young children,* San Diego, 1994, Singular.

Gibbon FE, Beck JM: Therapy for abnormal vowels in children with phonological impairment. In Ball MJ, Gibbon FE, editors: *Vowel disorders,* Boston, 2002, Butterworth-Heinemann.

Kent RD: *The speech sciences,* San Diego, 1997, Singular.

Ling D: *Speech and the hearing-impaired child: theory and practice,* Washington, DC, 1976, The Alexander Graham Bell Association for the Deaf and Hard of Hearing.

Ling D: *Speech and the hearing-impaired child: theory and practice,* ed 2, Washington, DC, 2002, The Alexander Graham Bell Association for the Deaf and Hard of Hearing.

Ling D, Ling AH: *Aural rehabilitation: the foundations of verbal learning in hearing-impaired children,* Washington, DC, 1978, The Alexander Graham Bell Association for the Deaf and Hard of Hearing.

Northern JL, Downs MP: *Hearing in children,* ed 5, Philadelphia, 2002, Lippincott Williams & Wilkins.

Owens RE Jr: *Language development: an introduction,* ed 6, Boston, 2005, Allyn & Bacon.

Paterson MM: Articulation and phonological disorders in hearing-impaired school-aged children with severe and profound sensorineural losses. In Bernthal J, Bankson N, editors: *Child phonology: characteristics, assessment, and intervention with special populations,* New York, 1994, Thieme Medical.

Perigoe CB: Strategies for the remediation of hearing-impaired children, *Volta Rev* 94:95-118, 2002.

Revoile SG: Hearing loss and the audibility of phoneme cues. In Pickett JM, editor: *The acoustics of speech communication,* Boston, 1999, Allyn & Bacon.

Robbins AM: Rehabilitation after cochlear implantation. In Niparko JK, Kirk KI, Mellon NK et al, editors: *Cochlear implants: principles and practices,* Philadelphia, 2000, Lippincott Williams & Wilkins.

Roberts JE, Clarke-Klein S: Otitis media. In Bernthal J, Bankson N, editors: *Child phonology: characteristics, assessment, and intervention,* New York, 1994, Thieme Medical.

Ross M, Brackett D, Maxon AB: *Assessment and management of mainstreamed hearing-impaired children: principles and practices,* Austin, Tex, 1991, Pro-Ed.

Shriberg LD, Kent RD: *Clinical phonetics,* ed 2, Boston, 1995, Allyn & Bacon.

Shriberg, LD, Friel-Patti, S, Flipsen, P et al: Otitis media, fluctuant hearing loss, and speech-language outcomes: a preliminary structural equation model, *J Speech Lang Hear Res* 43:100-120, 2000.

Tye-Murray N: *Foundations of aural rehabilitation: children, adults, and their family members,* ed 2, Clifton Park, NY, 2004, Delmar Learning.

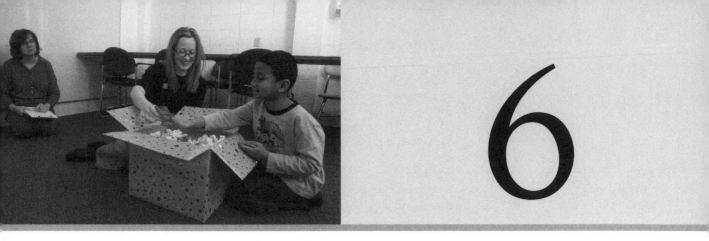

6

Alternative Treatments for Residual Errors

LEARNING GOALS
- Define residual errors.
- Identify at least one common and uncommon distortion error.
- Briefly describe the treatments used with children who have residual errors.
- Discuss biofeedback and speech appliances as forms of alternative treatment for children with sound system disorders. What do the data suggest about the efficacy of these methods?
- Identify several issues involved in the use of biofeedback and speech appliances.

In some cases, clients exhibit sound system errors beyond the age of expected developmental acquisition, which generally has an upper bound limit of 9 years of age. That is, they exhibit residual errors and the errors may persist into adulthood. Typically, individuals in this diagnostic entity have not responded to traditional treatments, or they have maintained the sound system error after expected developmental maturation. These clients, although few in number, often acquire correct production of target phonemes through the use of specialized treatments. These treatment options use principles of biofeedback to provide important information to the learner or attempt to develop appropriate place and manner of production through the use of speech appliances to position the articulators.

Although most individuals with sound system disorders undergo successful treatment, a subset of clients do not correct their problems. This population consists of children who do not respond to traditional treatments or who exhibit developmental errors that persist beyond the age of expected developmental acquisition. In some cases the individuals have sound system errors that continue into adulthood (Shriberg et al., 1994). These individuals require treatment because mastery of the phonological system is critical to language development, reading, and other academic areas (Shriberg and Kwiatkowski, 1994). In addition, Crowe Hall (1991) published a report that studied normal speakers' perceptions of children with sound system disorders and found that normal speakers react negatively to speakers with even minor sound system disorders. Moreover, negativity toward speakers with sound system disorders has been a consistent finding in the literature (Mowrer et al., 1978; Silverman and Paulus, 1989). To identify and treat this population, the speech-language pathologist must be aware of the category of residual errors and the treatments that may be applied to this population.

A published report that studied normal speakers' perceptions of children with sound system disorders found that normal speakers react negatively to speakers with even minor sound system errors.

Research Note

Crowe Hall, 1991.

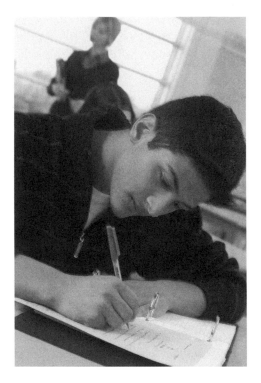

Mastery of the phonological system is critical to language development, reading, and other academic areas. Clients who do not respond to traditional treatments can exhibit residual errors if alternative means of treatment are not identified and implemented. (Copyright 2007, JupiterImages Corporation.)

RESIDUAL ERRORS

Residual errors are a subtype of sound system errors. These errors do not normalize with treatment or through maturation and continue past the expected period of speech sound acquisition for some clients (Shriberg, 1997). Residual errors are found in the speech of older school-aged children and adult speakers. Shriberg has further subdivided the group into those who were diagnosed with a speech delay and received treatment and those who did not receive such a diagnosis during the developmental period but exhibited errors that they maintained.

Most residual errors are classified as distortions of the intended phoneme and do not fall within the perceptual boundaries of that phoneme (Bernthal and Bankson, 2004; Daniloff et al., 1980; Ruscello, 2003). Shriberg (1993) indicates that the hypothesized causal agents for distortion errors may be permanent or temporary factors during speech development. Researchers postulate that **distortion errors** are the result of incorrect allophonic rules and/or sensorimotor processing limitations. That is, the child develops internally an incorrect production level rule that manifests in the distortion, or the child's sensorimotor control of surface productions is defective, resulting in the perceived distortion. According to Ohde and Sharf (1992), distortions have very distinctive physiologic and acoustic correlates that are characteristic of the nonallophonic variations. For example, a lateral lisp of /s/ is produced with the tongue tip in contact with the alveolus, and the airstream is directed off both sides (or one side) of the tongue. The acoustic result is a sound with lower intensity and frequency than /s/.

Distortion errors have very distinctive physiologic and acoustic correlates that are characteristic of the nonallophonic variations.	*Research* **Note**

Ohde and Sharf, 1992.

Box 6-1 presents a summary of common and uncommon distortion errors that have been described in the literature (Smit et al., 1990; Shriberg, 1993). As noted, the most frequent common distortions encompass the sound classes of fricatives, affricatives, and liquids. Ruscello (1995b) summarized survey data that had been collected from 98 speech-language pathologists who provided services to school-aged children. A majority of respondents indicated that a small proportion of their respective clients either failed to acquire correct production of a target sound or acquired production but failed to develop spontaneous production of the target. The most frequent phonemes listed were /r/, /s/, and /z/, which is in agreement with the data reported by Shriberg (1993). Generally the common distortions do not have a significant effect on intelligibility, but their existence does call attention to the speaker (Crowe Hall, 1991). The uncommon distortions are errors that are characteristic of system-wide production problems often seen in individuals with sound system disorders that are not developmental phonological disorders, but rather are symptomatic of structural, sensory, or motor involvement. For instance, clients with problems such as cleft lip and palate, hearing loss, and dysarthria may demonstrate system-wide distortion errors such as those listed as uncommon distortions. Moreover,

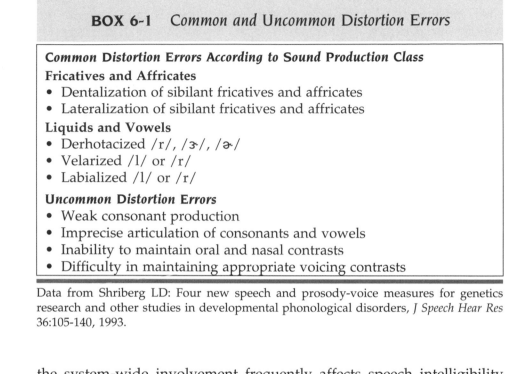

BOX 6-1   *Common and Uncommon Distortion Errors*

Common Distortion Errors According to Sound Production Class
Fricatives and Affricates
- Dentalization of sibilant fricatives and affricates
- Lateralization of sibilant fricatives and affricates

Liquids and Vowels
- Derhotacized /r/, /ɝ/, /ɚ/
- Velarized /l/ or /r/
- Labialized /l/ or /r/

Uncommon Distortion Errors
- Weak consonant production
- Imprecise articulation of consonants and vowels
- Inability to maintain oral and nasal contrasts
- Difficulty in maintaining appropriate voicing contrasts

Data from Shriberg LD: Four new speech and prosody-voice measures for genetics research and other studies in developmental phonological disorders, *J Speech Hear Res* 36:105-140, 1993.

the system-wide involvement frequently affects speech intelligibility negatively.

Research Note   A survey of 98 school speech-language pathologists indicated that a majority had a small proportion of children on their caseloads who either failed to acquire correct production of a target sound or acquired production but failed to develop spontaneous production of that target. The most frequent phonemes in error were /r/, /s/, and /z/.

Ruscello, 1995b.

TREATMENT

Treatment for children with residual errors typically consists of a motor skill–learning approach (Fletcher, 1992; Gierut, 1998), and many clients normalize their sound system errors with this treatment. The clients are first taught to acquire correct production of the target sound. After acquisition, practice activities are used to automate the target sound in a variety of different practice levels including spontaneous conversation (see Chapter 2). However, clients who do not acquire the target sound require specialized treatments that incorporate principles of **biofeedback** or use **speech appliances** to assist in acquisition and automatization of target phonemes (Ruscello, 2003). Basmajiam (1989) indicates that biofeedback has a history in the medical profession; it has been used for such problems as pain management and muscle reeducation. Specialists (e.g., prosthodontists) have constructed dental appliances to obturate structural defects and improve dental occlusion (Peterson-Falzone et al., 2001). However, in the current discussion, speech appliances are devices that are used to position the articulators and facilitate correct production of a target sound. The reader should note that an appliance positions an articulator in a specific position and cannot be used in connected speech because it restricts the movement of individual articulators (Clark et al., 1993).

An appliance positions an articulator in a specific position and cannot be used in connected speech because it restricts the movement of individual articulators.

Research Note

Clark et al., 1993.

Biofeedback

Biofeedback has been used extensively in the treatment of residual errors and other speech and swallowing disorders (Crary and Groher, 2000; McGuire, 1995; Volin, 1998). Performance information that generally is not available on a conscious level is provided so that the learner may modify his or her current performance. Davis and Drichta (1980) describe biofeedback in the following way:

> Specifically, biofeedback can be defined as the use of instrumentation to provide moment-to-moment information about a specific physiological system that is under control of the nervous system but not clearly or accurately perceived. Biofeedback derives its effectiveness by making ambiguous internal cues explicit, thereby providing accurate information about changes in target responses (i.e., muscle tension) during training so that instrumental control of the response is facilitated. By precisely detecting a physiological event and then converting the resulting electronic signal into auditory, visual, tactile, or kinesthetic feedback, a subject can be made immediately and continuously aware of the level of a physiological event. (p. 288)

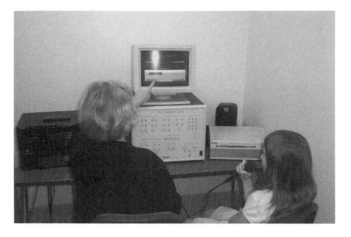

Figure 6-1 ■ Biofeedback in the form of acoustic information is being provided to this client. The clinician has produced a target item and is attempting to have the client match the target via visual biofeedback.

Biofeedback can take many forms, but applications in the literature for sound system disorders generally provide clients with immediate acoustic or physiologic performance signals (Bernhardt et al., 2005; Dagenais, 1995; Gibbon, 1999; Ruscello, 1995b). For example, a client can receive actual frequency and amplitude information pertaining to a target sound, or the signal could be transformed into some colorful display. Shriberg and colleagues (1990) categorize the latter software displays as either *iconic* or *thematic* in presentation. An iconic display exhibits changes in size or color as a function of variations in frequency and amplitude, whereas a thematic display consists of some type of game or other simulation that changes as a function of differing frequency and amplitude information. Most applications of **acoustic biofeedback** use the actual acoustic signal to modify target productions (Shuster et al., 1995). Figure 6-1 shows a client who is undegoing acoustic biofeedback.

Physiologic biofeedback is similar in terms of providing performance information, but the signals may differ according to the type of information (Bernhardt et al., 2005; Crary and Groher, 2000; Gibbon et al., 1999; Michi et al., 1993; Ruscello et al., 1991). For example, Ruscello and colleagues used a nasal airflow signal to treat an adult who exhibited phoneme-specific nasal emission for /s/. The subject was able to use the information and modify production of the /s/. After the sound

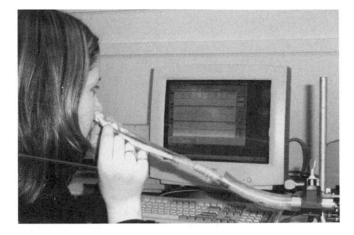

***Figure* 6-2** ■ An adult client is receiving visual biofeedback on generation of oral pressure and unwanted nasal airflow during the production of pressure sounds. Plosives, fricatives, and affricates require the generation of sufficient pressure for production.

was acquired, the biofeedback signal was withdrawn and automatization practice activities were introduced so that the sound was used in spontaneous conversation. In Figure 6-2, an adult client is undergoing visual biofeedback.

An investigation reported by Shuster and colleagues (1995) is another example of a biofeedback study that used acoustic information. The authors provided treatment to two adolescents with residual errors. A real-time **sound spectrograph** was used to display acoustic information, which initially contrasted the subject's errors with the investigator's correct production. After discussion of the differences in the productions, subjects were instructed to modify their displays to reflect correct sound production. Both subjects were successful and achieved correct production of target sounds despite long-term treatment using traditional methodologies. Similarly, Bernhardt and colleagues (2005) report the use of **ultrasound** in treating adolescents and adults with residual errors. The authors report the method permits clear visualization of different tongue shapes, and subjects are able to use the information when forming correct articulatory positions. Finally, Dagenais and associates (Dagenais, 1995; Dagenais et al., 1994) and Gibbon and her research group (Gibbon, 1999; Gibbon et al., 1999) have used **electropalatography** very extensively. Subjects are custom fitted with an acrylic hard

Table 6-1
Summary of Biofeedback Instruments

TYPE OF BIOFEEDBACK	SIGNAL
Acoustic	
Real-time sound spectrograph	Display of acoustic information
Physiologic	
Palatograph	Display of tongue palate contact
Ultrasound	Display of tongue articulations
Aerodynamics	Display of air pressure and/or airflow

palate that contains a series of electrodes leading to a processing unit and computer display. When tongue movement is initiated, location and timing of tongue and hard palate articulation is captured. The authors report success with a wide variety of subjects who have sound system disorders. Table 6-1 summarizes the different types of biofeedback used in the treatment of sound system errors.

Some practitioners may be intimidated by the use of biofeedback instrumentation, because many do not have the necessary expertise to operate the equipment or do not have ready access to equipment. As discussed previously, a motor skill approach is used to achieve production—practice may encompass isolated sounds, syllables, words, phrases, sentences, and conversation. However, the initial components of the biofeedback process are designed to create a mental focus on the target so that the client may use the information to acquire correct target sound production and practice the target within the principles of motor skill learning. Ruscello (1995b) proposed that the biofeedback treatment model is a cognitive-based process that involves introspection and analysis on the part of the client.

Research Note	Biofeedback treatment has been described as a cognitive-based process that involves introspection and analysis on the part of the client.

Ruscello, 1995b.

BOX 6-2   *Common Elements of a Biofeedback Treatment Model*

Schema

1. Clinician produces examples of the desired target and displays the biofeedback information to the client.
2. Clinician describes the production features of the target sound for the client.
3. Clinician contrasts the desired target production with the client's production.
4. Client is instructed to focus mentally on the task and attempt to match the correct target using biofeedback information so that acquisition occurs.
5. Results of practice trials are evaluated.
   • Client self-evaluation and feedback
   • Clinician evaluation of practice and knowledge of results
6. Practice is continued without biofeedback to automate the target sound.

The basic elements of a biofeedback model are summarized in Box 6-2. Initially the client is introduced to the biofeedback process. The clinician produces the target sound and discusses the biofeedback display with the client. The information that is displayed is only available via biofeedback; consequently, the client must be oriented to the signal. The clinician also explains the production features of the target sound while furnishing examples of the target sound. The first two steps are then followed by a contrast stage wherein examples of the target sound are contrasted with the client's error production. This process enables the client to observe differences between the model and the current production.

The next step is a production step that involves the client attempting to modify his or her current production by using the biofeedback. This step requires mental focus on the part of the client because he or she must use the information to change production characteristics. Gibbon and colleagues (1999) stated, "The use of biofeedback in treatment derives its effectiveness from making ambiguous internal cues explicit . . . and enabling conscious control of such cues to develop." Client and clinician evaluation and discussion of results follow each practice trial; both performance feedback and knowledge of results are available to the learner. The goal is to develop a correspondence between the acoustic or physiologic information and resultant perceptual output. That is, when the client produces a target with the appropriate acoustic or physiologic match, a corresponding perceptual match exists. The client has developed the orosensory information requisite to correct sound production (Ertmer et al., 1996). After acquisition of the target has been achieved, the biofeedback technique is faded in favor of traditional treatment and automatization of the target sound in spontaneous speaking contexts.

CASE STUDY 6-1

Visual Biofeedback: A Phonetic Approach to Treatment with Residual Errors

D.S. is a 12-year-old girl who misarticulated the consonant /r/ and the vocalic variants /ɝ, ɚ/. The client received 4 years of traditional phonetic treatment for /r/, with no success before the current testing. The residual errors were described perceptually as distortions of the intended target sounds. Contextual testing did not identify any variants of the targets that were identified as perceptually correct. No other sound system errors were noted, and intelligibility was within normal limits; however, the /r/ misarticulations were perceptually distinctive to the examiner. The client also reported that peers would sometimes identify the /r/ errors when conversing with her. An oral mechanism screening was within normal limits, as was hearing acuity for pure tones.

The client was enrolled for 10 weekly 50-minute sessions in a treatment program that used biofeedback to achieve correct production of /r/ and the vocalic variants. Biofeedback provides the learner with performance information that is generally not available on a conscious level. A Kay Elemetrics Model 5500 real-time spectrograph was used to provide the client with a visual acoustic record of performance. The biofeedback treatment consisted of three phases of treatment, which included an introductory phase, identification phase, and production phase. Initially the clinician articulated a number of different vowel sounds and had the client listen and observe the acoustic information that was displayed on the spectrograph. Formant structure of the different vowels was identified for the client as "bunches or groupings of sound energy," and each distinctive pattern was illustrated.

When the client could identify the formant structure correctly in 8 of 10 consecutive trials of different vowel presentations, the introductory phase was terminated. This was followed by an identification phase, in which the clinician produced tokens of /ɝ/ and /r/, paused the spectrograph, and then had the client produce a practice token. The clinician's token and the client's token were displayed together so that the clinician could compare and contrast the practice tokens in terms of formant structure. In particular, the merging of F2 and F3 was distinguished for the client as an important visual cue that was associated with correct /r/ production. The identification phase was terminated after the client was able to identify differences between her practice tokens and those of the clinician in 8 of 10 consecutive trials. The first two phases were completed in a single practice session.

The production phase involved practice of /ɝ/, /ir/, and /ar/ by the client. D.S. was seated in front of the spectrograph and produced a practice token. A response was judged to be correct if the clinician judged it to be perceptually correct and if the acoustic representation exhibited an acoustic formant pattern that was consistent with correct /r/ production. Practice was intense, with the client producing between 125 and 150 practice tokens per session. At the termination of the biofeedback treatment, D.S. was capable of producing the /r/ and vocalic variants correctly. Practice then shifted to production of the target sounds in words, phrases, sentences, and spontaneous speech, without the visual biofeedback information.

Commentary

D.S. had a residual error that was resistant to traditional treatment. It was necessary to introduce biofeedback information so that the client could acquire correct production of consonant /r/ and the vocalic variants /ɝ, ɚ/. The client was required to focus mentally on the treatment task while receiving sensory feedback, including the addition of visual acoustic information. This was also supplemented with KR (knowledge of results) from the clinician. Once acquisition had occurred, motor skill–learning techniques were introduced to facilitate automatization of the targets in different contexts.

Evaluation of Biofeedback Treatment

Research data support biofeedback as a viable treatment for residual errors that are resistant to correction through traditional methods. Volin (1998) conducted a selected review of biofeedback studies in the literature that dealt with different speech disorders. Within the group of studies, seven treatment studies involved sound system disorders. Three of the investigations treated children with errors of unknown cause, three studied children with hearing impairment, and a single study dealt with children born with cleft palate. Positive results were reported in all cases; however, most studies were individual or small group case studies that examined the effectiveness of biofeedback in a single-subject, repeated-measures design without a nonbiofeedback comparison group. In terms of evidence-based practice, further empiric scrutiny is needed because a valid treatment must be grounded in the highest degree of scientific rigor (Baker and McLeod, 2004; Clark, 2005; Justice and Fey, 2004: Lass et al., 2004). Credible evidence supports biofeedback as a treatment for children with sound system errors who are resistant to traditional treatment, but further empiric evidence is needed.

Research Note	In a selected review of biofeedback studies, seven treatment studies were found to involve sound system disorders: three that treated children with errors of unknown cause, three that studied children with hearing impairment, and one that dealt with children born with cleft palate. In all cases the efficacy of biofeedback was substantiated.

Volin, 1998.

One may ask why some clients experience difficulty with the acquisition of certain phonemes and develop production errors that are frequently resistant to traditional therapies. As mentioned previously, distortion errors may be the result of incorrect allophonic rules or sensorimotor processing limitations. Biofeedback researchers have explained their data in relation to either of the two hypotheses. Shuster and colleagues (Shuster et al., 1992; Shuster et al., 1995) offer a hypothesis that is aligned with the incorrect allophonic rules explanation. Their explanation posits that the underlying representation of the phoneme is defective. That is, a speaker of the language has underlying representations of individual morphemes. The underlying representation is an abstract account that includes a semantic component and the learned phonological characteristics of the morpheme. In addition, some researchers speculate that the child has both receptive and expressive representations of morphemes. The **receptive representation** includes the auditory features of words that the child can understand, whereas the **expressive representation** contains the articulatory features of the words that the child can produce. According to Straight (1980), receptive and expressive representations are independent of each other, but they may influence each other. As the child's phonology develops, a merging of the receptive and expressive levels of representation occurs. The child with a residual error may have failed to merge the receptive and expressive representations. In this case, he or she will not benefit from a traditional treatment paradigm that uses auditory stimuli because they do not have an internal model of the correct target phoneme.

Why do some clients have difficulty acquiring certain phonemes and develop production errors that are frequently resistant to traditional therapy? One hypothesis posits that the underlying representation of the phoneme is defective.

Research Note

Shuster et al., 1995.

Researchers hypothesize that receptive and expressive representations of a phoneme are independent but may influence each other as a child's phonology develops.

Research Note

Straight, 1980.

A hypothesis formulated by Gibbon (1999) suggests that residual errors can be explained as a motor control deficit. Gibbon and other researchers (Dagenais, 1995) have analyzed electropalatography tracings of school-aged children with sound system disorders and identified lingual and palate contacts that they have labeled as *undifferentiated gestures*. The key feature of undifferentiated gestures is anterior midsagittal and posterior midsagittal lingual and palate contact during the production of anterior lingual sounds. This place of articulation differs from the typical lingual and palate contact seen in the productions of normal-speaking children. Gibbon speculates that undifferentiated gestures are markers of either delayed or disordered motor control. The delay hypothesis implies that undifferentiated gestures are present in the normal child's articulatory development because they are a reflection of a motor control system that is maturing. Conversely, the disordered hypothesis suggests that undifferentiated gestures are compensatory strategies that do not solve the production needs of the speaker; therefore developmental errors habituate and become residual errors.

Research Note	An alternative hypothesis suggests that residual errors can be explained as a motor control deficit. Undifferentiated gestures (atypical lingual and palatal contacts) are thought to be markers of either delayed or disordered motor control.

Gibbon, 1999.

Speech Appliances

As defined earlier, the term *speech appliance*—in the context of this discussion—is a device that is used to position the articulators for the purpose of establishing correct production of a target sound (Box 6-3). It differs from biofeedback in that the client is not given some abstract physiologic signal. A history exists of the devices or appliances being used for positioning the articulators, and the appliances range from very crude devices such as modified tongue blades and wooden dowels to custom-fabricated devices (Borden, 1974, 1984). For example, Altshuler (1961) describes the construction of a device for positioning the articulators to produce the /s/ speech sound. The clinician modifies a **tongue blade** by cutting a piece approximately 30 mm in length and then making an angle cut of approximately 25 degrees at the cut end. The wedge-shaped device is placed in contact with the tongue in the vertical plane and centered in midline. The shape and position of the modified tongue blade is said to prevent lateralization and promote a central airstream

---

BOX 6-3   *Examples of Speech Appliances*

- *Modified tongue blade*—wedge-shaped device that places the tongue in contact with the vertical plane and centered in midline; helps the client produce the /s/ sound.
- *Prosthetic placement cues*—oral appliance used inside or outside the oral cavity to help the client position the articulators to produce an intended target sound; helps the client produce the /r/ sound.
- *Wooden dowel*—device inserted in the side of the mouth in contact with the upper and lower molar surfaces to stabilize the mandible; helps the client position the tongue in place to produce /r/.
- *Custom dental appliances*—device constructed by a dentist and inserted into the maxillary arch, similar to an orthodontic retainer; held in place by dental clasps to help position the client's tongue to produce /r/.

requisite to /s/ production. The author indicates that 9 of 10 subjects acquired correct production of the target sound in isolation when the device was placed in contact with the tongue. Transfer of the sound to contextual stimuli was achieved by instructing the subjects to "imagine" that the appliance was still positioning their tongue for /s/ in isolation.

Mowrer (1970) notes that some clients require what he refers to as "prosthetic placement cues" to attain correct target sound production. The **prosthetic placement cues** consist of some type of oral appliance that is used outside or inside the oral cavity for the purpose of positioning the articulators to produce the intended target sound. Mowrer discusses the development of a device to position the articulators for the purpose of eliciting the /r/ sound. The device is a small plastic plate that inserts under the tongue and creates a lingual place of articulation that is conducive to production of /r/. The success rate with the device is not mentioned, but the author indicates that clients with /r/ errors are able to achieve perceptually correct sounds. The appliance cannot be used for contextual practice of /r/. Similarly, a case study discussed by Leonti and colleagues (1975) describes a client who did not acquire correct /r/ production through traditional treatment. The clinicians fabricated an oral speech appliance that was inserted in the mouth to position the tongue for correct sound placement. The authors report that the client was able to attain correct production of the /r/ in isolation with the device in place.

A report by Shriberg (1980) does not include the use of an appliance to elicit /r/, but he uses a **wooden dowel** that is inserted in the side of the mouth. The dowel is in contact with the upper and lower molar surfaces to stabilize the mandible so that the client may position the tongue in place to produce /r/. The author describes the procedure in the following way:

> Do not give any instructions to the child, but rather let the child try to understand that the tongue by itself can produce good vowels or semi-vowels . . . or good /r/. . . . On their own, children seem to "get it." The clinician sits back continuing calmly to model the correct sound, refraining from all directions about tongue or lip placement. The mirror is handy to show the contrast between relaxed lips and overly rounded lips, but let the child take the lead. Encourage the child to find for himself or herself the tongue posture that produces a sound that matches the clinician's model. (p. 109)

The jaw stabilization is withdrawn when the client can produce perceptually correct /r/ in the context of CV syllables. The author reports that stabilization of the jaw with the wooden dowel was successful for a group of approximately 12 clients. Shriberg (1980) reports that stabilization of the jaw helps create conscious awareness of tongue position without the interference of lip and jaw movements. The use of a dowel is similar to the use of a bite block for the purpose of jaw stabilization (see Chapter 3).

The final study in this series was carried out by Clark and colleagues (1993) and also dealt with acquisition of /r/. The researchers developed an appliance **(prosthesis)** that inserted in the maxillary arch similar to an orthodontic retainer. The appliances were constructed by a dentist and custom made for each child. The appliance was held in place by dental clasps and positioned the tongue for production of /r/. Clark and colleagues recruited a group of 36 subjects who met certain criteria including traditional /r/ treatment for at least 6 months with no significant change. The subjects were randomly assigned to one of four groups, which included the appliance and auditory stimulation during treatment, the appliance and no auditory stimulation, no appliance but auditory stimulation, and no appliance and no auditory stimulation. The auditory stimulation consisted of the clinician's imitative modeling of the target sound at each practice level. The nonauditory stimulation condition had the clinician provide placement cues but no auditory models of /r/. All subjects were given opportunities to practice the target sound at the isolation, syllable, and word levels. Statistical analysis indicated that children in both appliance groups demonstrated statistically higher scores than children in the nonappliance groups. The researchers felt that the statistical difference was the result of the appliance groups' ability to achieve almost immediate success with isolated /r/ and the ability to practice /r/ in context earlier than the nonappliance groups.

Evaluation of Speech Appliances and Devices

The data discussed herein indicate that appliances and devices have a place in the modification of sound system errors. In the case of residual errors that are resistant to traditional treatment, positioning the articulators does assist the learner in acquiring correct placement. Researchers believe that it provides the client with sensory feedback that he or she may use to develop correct production and enable the appliance to be removed without a decrement in performance (Ruscello, 1995a). One needs to be cognizant of the fact that something is inserted in the mouth and thus limits production capabilities, because clients cannot engage in spontaneous speech with a positioning appliance inserted in the mouth. The appliances resulted in correct production of the target sound. How does one account for the positive performance change with the appliance in place? The speakers may have reacted to the alteration in oral anatomy by modifying their speech motor control rules while guided by the goal of producing perceptually correct speech.

When residual errors are resistant to treatment, positioning of the articulators may help the client acquire correct placement. Researchers believe that this provides the client with sensory feedback that can be used to develop correct production, enabling eventual removal of the appliance without a loss of performance.

Research Note

Ruscello, 1995a.

Moon and Jones (1991) hypothesize that the interactive relationship among speech articulators is one of coordinative structures that have the primary goal of developing perceptually correct speech under different speaking conditions. The articulators such as the lips, jaw, and tongue interact during speech production, but the contributions of each articulator may differ according to a specific speaking context or other unpredictable conditions. The differential contributions of the articulators in achieving a motor goal are reflective of a coordinative structure synergy. Speakers develop broad motor rules that are not at the individual phone level; rather, they are holistic rules that are tied to the speaker's message. Degrees of freedom exist in which the articulators may interact to produce perceptually correct speech. The speakers in the studies formed correct sounds with the appliance in place, suggesting that they modified motor rules to accommodate production of the target sound. After achieving correct production with the appliance, it was removed; however, speakers maintained correct production because the appropriate articulatory movements became incorporated into their existing rule system.

IDENTIFYING AT-RISK CLIENTS

The different methods discussed earlier have been used with a limited number of clients who experienced problems in the acquisition and/or automatization of one or more speech sounds. In examining the studies, it is important to identify common factors that may be associated with clients who may be at risk for sound system learning through traditional treatment methods. In most cases it was an acquisition problem, and the /r/ phoneme was the target of treatment. The literature is replete with references to production deficiencies associated with /r/ production (Creaghead and Newman, 1989). In addition, the sound system errors were frequently described as distortion errors. The reader should recall that distortion errors are productions that are not within the perceptual boundaries of the intended phoneme (Daniloff et al., 1980).

In most studies, subjects received traditional treatment that ranged from 6 months to approximately 2 years, and it was reported that they failed to demonstrate significant gains after the periods of treatment. In addition, the lack of stimulability in older clients may also be an indicator that traditional treatment methods may be ineffective. Volin (1998) carried out a motor-learning experiment that had normal subjects learn to control breathing rate during quiet breathing. A baseline condition was used to identify the subjects' stimulability for the task, and they were randomly assigned to either a biofeedback treatment group or a verbal feedback treatment group. The results of the study indicated that subjects with poor stimulability showed significantly more improvement if assigned to the biofeedback treatment, not the verbal feedback treatment. The author concluded that biofeedback should be considered as an option in cases wherein a client exhibits poor stimulability for a task during baseline evaluation or trial treatment. These findings suggest that practitioners must be alert to such clients so that they may consider other treatment options with the client and caregivers. Table 6-2 summarizes the risk factors identified.

Table 6-2
Common Factors Associated with the Use of Alternative Sound System Error Treatment

FACTOR	CLIENT RISK FACTOR
Type of sound system error	Most likely a distortion error, which is not within the perceptual boundaries of the intended phoneme
Level of treatment breakdown	Failure to acquire correct target sound production
Duration of treatment	Six months or more of treatment without success
Trial stimulability	Not stimulable for target during initial trial therapy

In one experiment, normal subjects were asked to learn to control breathing rate during quiet breathing; these subjects were randomly assigned to either a biofeedback treatment group or a verbal feedback treatment group. Results indicated that individuals with poor stimulability showed significantly more improvement if they were assigned to the biofeedback group.	*Research Note*

Volin, 1998.

FEASIBILITY OF USING BIOFEEDBACK OR SPEECH APPLIANCES

Biofeedback procedures and speech appliances are methods that have been used for a small subset of clients with sound system disorders, and the results have been very positive. However, issues regarding the general feasibility of the methods are discussed in this chapter (Box 6-4). For instance, treatment via acoustic or physiologic biofeedback requires instrumentation to provide an appropriate signal to the client. Instrumentation costs have diminished in the past years, and software has been developed for a variety of computer operating systems (Gibbon and Beck, 2002; Masterson and Rvachew, 1999; McGuire, 1995). However, costs must still be considered, particularly when the clinician

---

BOX 6-4   *Issues Surrounding the Use of Biofeedback and Speech Appliances*

Drawbacks
- Instrumentation costs
- Impracticality (e.g., too much time and effort)
- Custom-made palatal plates for electropalatography
- Dental fabrication
- Sophisticated level of clinician experience

Opportunities
- Cooperative service delivery model to combine resources of two or more facilities
- Center-based model in which clinicians refer clients to regional centers
- Generic appliance development for use by any number of clients

must justify the purchase of instrumentation for a limited number of clients. In addition, some equipment such as ultrasound would not be practical in most treatment entities, and electropalatography requires the construction of custom-made palatal plates. Similarly, the speech appliance developed by Clark and associates (1993) requires fabrication of the appliance by a dentist. Finally, the use of instrumentation requires a certain level of sophistication that some practitioners may not have.

Although a number of issues were identified that preclude the widespread use of alternative treatments, opportunities exist for their use with clients who have sound system disorders. For example, Ruscello and colleagues (1995) developed a cooperative service delivery model between a university clinic and local school system. The client attended the university clinic for biofeedback treatment that enabled him to acquire correct target sound production. When this stage of treatment was completed, the school speech-language pathologist conducted automatization activities at the client's school. The case study is an example of two facilities working in cooperative fashion to treat a client who needed an alternative form of remediation. Gibbon and colleagues (1999) use electropalatography extensively with children who need alternative treatments for sound system disorders. The researchers report the development of regional centers in their country where practitioners may refer clients for electropalatography treatment. The center-based model provides treatment opportunities for clients who previously were unable to receive such services because of geographic locale and financial cost.

| Research Note | In one cooperative service delivery model, the client attended a university clinic for biofeedback treatment and later followed up with the school-based speech-language pathologist for automatization activities. In another model, regional centers were developed where clinicians could refer clients for electropalatography treatment. In a third model, clients who met certain criteria were fitted with appliances at a university clinic, but were treated at the client's school by a local practitioner. |

Clark et al., 1993; Gibbon et al., 1999; Ruscello et al., 1995.

Clark and colleagues (1993) also used a cooperative model and informed practitioners that clients who met certain sound system characteristics could receive a speech appliance that might facilitate correct production of the /r/. The children were fitted with the appliances at a university medical center; however, the local practitioner conducted all treatment at the client's school. Clark's model embodies the cooperative treatment feature reported by Ruscello and colleagues (1995) and the regional availability feature discussed by Gibbon and colleagues (1999). A final consideration in the development of speech appliances might be the fabrication of a generic appliance that could be used by any number of clients. It could be sterilized and used repeatedly by a practitioner when needed.

SUMMARY

A small group of children who experience sound system errors do not respond to traditional treatment. These children display residual errors, which are generally classified perceptually as *distortion errors*. A number of studies reported in the literature have successfully modified residual sound system errors using various forms of biofeedback or speech appliances to position the articulators. Researchers have proposed different hypothesizes to explain why clients develop residual errors, as well as why the errors are resistant to traditional therapy. A number of risk factors appear to be characteristic of this group. The characteristics include the presence of distortion errors, failure to acquire correct production of the target sound, significant amounts of treatment without positive gains, and lack of stimulability for the target.

Issues exist that restrict the widespread use of alternative treatments, such as those discussed in this chapter. However, some models of service provision have the potential to reach clients who need such services.

REFERENCES

Altshuler MW: A therapeutic oral device for lateral emission, *J Speech Hear Disord* 26:179-181, 1961.

Baker E, McLeod S: Evidence-based management of phonological impairment in children, *Child Lang Teach Ther* 20:261-285, 2004.

Basmajian JV: Introduction: principles and background. In Basmajian R, editor: *Biofeedback: principles and practice for clinicians,* Baltimore, 1989, Williams & Wilkins.

Bernhardt B, Gick B, Bacsfalvi P et al: Ultrasound in speech therapy with adolescents and adults, *Clin Linguist Phon* 19:605-617, 2005.

Bernthal JE, Bankson NW: *Articulation and phonological disorders,* ed 5, Boston, 2004, Allyn & Bacon.

Borden GJ: What is an orthophoniste? *ASHA* 16:203-206, 1974.

Borden GJ: Consideration of motor-sensory targets and problem of perception. In Winitz H, editor: *Treating articulation disorders: for clinicians by clinicians*, Austin, Tex, 1984, Pro-Ed.

Clark HM: Clinical decision making and oral motor treatments, *ASHA* 10:8-9, 34-35, 2005.

Clark CE, Schwarz IE, Blakeley RW: The removable r-appliance as a practice device to facilitate correct production of /r/, *Am J Speech Lang Pathol* 2:84-92, 1993.

Crary MA, Groher ME: Basic concepts of surface electromyographic biofeedback in the treatment of dysphagia: a tutorial, *Am J Speech Lang Pathol* 9:116-125, 2000.

Creaghead NA, Newman PW: Articulation and phonetics and phonology. In Creaghead NA, Newman PA, Secord WA, editors: *Assessment and remediation of articulatory and phonological disorders*, ed 2, Columbus, Ohio, 1989, Merrill.

Crowe Hall BJ: Attitudes of fourth and sixth graders toward peers with mild articulation disorders, *Lang Speech Hear Serv Sch* 22:334-339, 1991.

Dagenais PA: Electropalatography in the treatment of articulation/phonological disorders, *J Commun Disord* 28:303-330, 1995.

Dagenais PA, Critz-Crosby P, Adams JB: Comparing abilities of hearing-impaired children to learn consonants using palatographic or traditional aura-oral techniques, *J Speech Hear Res* 37:687-699, 1994.

Daniloff R, Wilcox K, Stephens MI: An acoustic-articulatory description of children's defective /s/ productions, *J Commun Disord* 13:347-363, 1980.

Davis SM, Drichta CE: Biofeedback: theory and application to speech pathology. In Lass N, editor: *Speech and language advances in basic research and practice*, New York, 1980, Academic Press.

Ertmer DJ, Stark RE, Karlan GR: Real-time spectrographic displays in vowel production training with children who have profound hearing loss, *Am J Speech Lang Pathol* 5:4-16, 1996.

Fletcher SG: *Articulation: a physiological approach*, San Diego, 1992, Singular.

Gibbon FE: Undifferentiated lingual gestures in children with articulatory phonological disorders, *J Speech Lang Hear Res* 42:382-397, 1999.

Gibbon FE, Beck JM: Therapy for abnormal vowels in children with phonological impairment. In Ball MJ, Gibbon FE, editors: *Vowel disorders*, Boston, 2002, Butterworth-Heinemann.

Gibbon FE, Stewart F, Hardcastle WJ et al: Widening access to electropalatography for children with persistent sound system disorders, *Am J Speech Lang Pathol* 8:319-334, 1999.

Gierut JA: Treatment efficacy: functional phonological disorders in children, *J Speech Lang Hear Res* 41(suppl):S85-S100, 1998.

Justice LM, Fey ME: Evidence-based practice in schools, *ASHA* 9:4-5, 2004.

Lass NJ, Ruscello DM, Pannbacker M: *Oral motor treatment in clinical speech-language pathology*. Proceedings of the American Speech-Language-Hearing Association Telephone Seminar, February 2004.

Leonti SL, Blakeley RW, Louis HM: *Spontaneous correction of resistant /r/ using an oral prosthesis.* Paper presented at the annual meeting of the American Speech-Language-Hearing Association, Washington, DC, 1975.

Masterson JJ, Rvachew S: Use of technology in phonological intervention, *Semin Speech Lang* 20:233-249, 1999.

McGuire RA: Computer-based instrumentation: issues in clinical applications, *Lang Speech Hear Serv Sch* 26:223-231, 1995.

Michi K, Yamashita Y, Satoko I et al: Role of visual feedback treatment for defective /s/ sounds in patients with cleft palate, *J Speech Hear Res* 36:277-285, 1993.

Moon JB, Jones DL: Motor control of velopharyngeal structures during vowel production, *Cleft Palate Craniofac J* 28:267-273, 1991.

Mowrer DE: *Lectures in methods of speech therapy,* Tempe, Ariz, 1970, Arizona State University Bookstore.

Mowrer DE, Wahl P, Doolan SJ: Effect of lisping on audience evaluation of male speakers, *J Speech Hear Disord* 43:140-148, 1978.

Ohde RN, Sharf DJ: *Phonetic analysis of normal and abnormal speech,* New York, 1992, Macmillan.

Peterson-Falzone SJ, Hardin-Jones MA, Karnell M: *Cleft palate speech,* ed 3, St Louis, 2001, Mosby.

Ruscello DM: Speech appliances in the treatment of phonological disorders, *J Commun Disord* 28:331-353, 1995a.

Ruscello DM: Visual feedback in treatment of residual phonological disorders, *J Commun Disord* 28:279-302, 1995b.

Ruscello DM: Residual phonological errors. In Kent R, editor: *Encyclopedia of communication disorders,* Boston, 2003, MIT Press.

Ruscello DM, Shuster LI, Sandwisch A: Modification of context-specific nasal emission, *J Speech Hear Res* 34:27-32, 1991.

Ruscello DM, Yanero D, Ghalichebaf M: Cooperative service delivery between a university clinic and a school system, *Lang Speech Hear Serv Sch* 26:273-277, 1995.

Shriberg LD: An intervention procedure for children with persistent /r/ errors, *Lang Speech Hear Serv Sch* 11:102-110, 1980.

Shriberg LD: Four new speech and prosody-voice measures for genetics research and other studies in developmental phonological disorders, *J Speech Hear Res* 36:105-140, 1993.

Shriberg LD: Developmental phonological disorders: one or many? In Hodson BW, Edwards ML, editors: *Perspectives in applied phonology,* Gaithersburg, Md, 1997, Aspen.

Shriberg LD, Gruber FA, Kwiatkowski J: Developmental phonological disorders III: long-term speech-sound normalization, *J Speech Hear Res* 37:1151-1177, 1994.

Shriberg LD, Kwiatkowski J: Developmental phonological disorders I: a clinical profile, *J Speech Hear Res* 37:1100-1126, 1994.

Shriberg LD, Kwiatkowski J, Snyder T: Tabletop versus microcomputer-assisted speech management: response evocation phase, *J Speech Hear Disord* 55:635-655, 1990.

Shuster LI, Ruscello DM, Smith KD: Evoking /r/ using visual feedback, *Am J Speech Lang Pathol* 1:29-34, 1992.

Shuster LI, Ruscello DM, Toth AR: The use of visual feedback to elicit correct /r/, *Am J Speech Lang Pathol* 4:37-44, 1995.

Silverman FH, Paulus PG: Peer reactions to teenagers who substitute /w/ for /r/, *Lang Speech Hear Serv Sch* 20:219-221, 1989.

Smit AB, Hand L, Freilinger JJ et al: The Iowa articulation norms project and its Nebraska replication, *J Speech Hear Disord* 55:779-798, 1990.

Straight HSS: Auditory versus articulatory phonological processes and their development in children. In Yeni-Komshian GH, Kavanagh JF, Ferguson CA, editors: *Child phonology volume 1: production,* New York, 1980, Academic Press.

Volin RA: A relationship between stimulability and the efficacy of visual feedback in the training of a respiratory control task, *Am J Speech Lang Pathol* 7:81-90, 1998.

Glossary

acoustic biofeedback   Provision of feedback to the learner in the form of some acoustic signal that is typically not available on a conscious level. The acoustic parameters of frequency, intensity, and duration (or a combination of these parameters) may be used to modify speech performance (see also *biofeedback*).

affricates   Class of consonant speech sounds that combine the production features of stops and fricatives. A complete closure of the vocal tract occurs, followed by a gradual release at the point of articulation. Examples are /tʃ/ and /dʒ/.

alveolar fricatives   Fricatives produced at the alveolar point of articulation (see also *fricatives*). Examples are /s, z/.

amplification   Process used to increase the intensity of sound.

ankyloglossia   Insertion and position of the lingual frenum is thought to restrict lingual movement. The anatomic condition is also referred to as *tongue-tie*.

antecedent events   Activities consisting of stimuli designed to elicit specific responses from a client during treatment.

antiresonances   Opposite of resonances or spectral peaks, because they are minima in the spectral envelope. Antiresonances are found in the production of nasal sounds because of the addition of a side branch (oral cavity) to the main resonating cavity (pharynx and nasal cavity).

articulatory knowledge   Client's knowledge of the production features of sounds (see also *phonological knowledge*).

ataxic dysarthria   Motor speech disorder caused by lesions to the cerebellar connections that link with the cortex. The major perceptual speech features are excess and equal stress problems (prosody) and imprecise consonant production.

audition   Process of hearing.

back vowels   Vowel sounds produced with the back or dorsum of the tongue (see also *vowels*). A number of back vowels are also produced with lip rounding.

basal ganglia   Group of nuclei located at the base of the cerebral hemispheres. Also known as the *extrapyramidal system*, these nuclei play a key role in the initiation and control of movement.

Beckwith-Wiedemann syndrome   Syndrome that may include growth; craniofacial, gastrointestinal, metabolic, genital, and motor development; and central nervous system involvement. Speech disorders are generally obligatory as a result of macroglossia and dental malocclusion.

bilabials   Speech sounds produced by articulation of the upper and lower lips. Examples include the speech sounds /b, p, m/.

biofeedback   Use of instrumentation to provide immediate information about a physiologic system that is under nervous system control but not clearly or accurately recognized by the learner.

bite block   Acrylic block placed in the side of the mouth between the teeth and designed to stabilize the jaw during speech treatment.

block sequencing   Motor learning concept that pertains to the administration of different levels of a treatment. The levels of the treatment are introduced in progression from less complex linguistically to more complex. This concept generally results in higher response accuracy levels during training trials but poorer generalization when compared with random sequencing.

capability-focus construct   Hypothetical treatment model that refers to the capacity or potential of the child for speech change as determined through assessment of phonology, consideration of any presenting risk factors, and the learning requisites of attention, motivation, and effort.

carrier sentence   Stereotypic sentence frame used to practice target sounds in the context of sentences.

childhood apraxia of speech (CAS)   Developmental motor speech disorder that is defined as a neurologic deficit involving the planning and programming of skilled movement requisite for speech production. The major features are sound production errors and prosodic variation.

cleft lip and palate   Birth defect that involves a lack of fusion of the lip, the palate, or both during prenatal development. These defects manifest in different degrees and variations of lip or palate involvement (or in different degrees and variations of both).

cognates   Sound pair in which each has the same place and manner of articulation but differs in relation to the presence or absence of laryngeal voicing. An example is the cognate pair /p, b/.

cognitive-linguistic variables   Variables such as intelligence, language, and academic performance that may function as causal correlates and coexist with sound system disorders.

compensatory errors   Sound system errors such as glottal stops that are used in substitution of intended speech sounds or speech sound classes. They are frequently found in the speech of children with velopharyngeal closure deficits or palatal fistulae.

conductive hearing loss   Difficulty with sound transmission caused by a problem that may exist anywhere from the external auditory canal up to the inner ear.

consequent events   Reinforcement or feedback contingencies that follow an individual's response to a stimulus.

contextual facilitation   Method that involves the probing of phonetic environments to identify the client's target productions that are perceived as being produced correctly.

continuous positive airway pressure (CPAP)   Procedure that can be used in therapeutic intervention for velopharyngeal closure deficits. Instrumentation is designed to furnish muscle resistance training during speech practice tasks.

contrastive drills   Therapy technique used in the treatment of developmental dysarthria. Contrasts among different word pairs are used to assist the client in developing distinctions among manner, place, or voicing problems (or a combination of these problems).

contrastive stress practice   Intervention technique used with clients who have dysarthria. The client produces an utterance but varies the prosodic pattern of the utterance in response to different clinician prompts.

control behavior   Behavior is independent from a behavior that is subject to treatment. Control behavior is periodically sampled during treatment and not expected to change, because the behavior is not being treated and is dissimilar in some way to the behavior being treated. This is often a component in single-subject design and is used to validate a treatment effect.

crossbite   Dental condition in which the maxillary teeth are inside or lingual to the mandibular teeth. The condition may vary from mild to severe.

cul-de-sac technique   Therapy technique used with children who have velopharyngeal closure deficits. The clinician or child occludes the child's nostrils to eliminate nasal air emission during the production of pressure sounds.

deaf   Profound hearing loss with an average hearing level of greater than 70 dB.

delayed auditory feedback (DAF)   Instrumentation is used to delay the auditory reception of one's speech. DAF is used with some clients to alter speaking rate for different speech disorders.

dental occlusion   Relationship between the upper and lower dental arches. The point of reference is the position of the upper and lower first molars.

developmental dysarthria   Motor speech disorder of sensorimotor execution. Children with this disorder exhibit difficulties in the execution of articulatory movements and possibly other components of speech production such as respiration, phonation, resonation, and prosody because of central or peripheral nervous system damage.

developmental errors   Normal variations found in the speech of children who are acquiring the sound system of their language. Because these sound errors are not a function of variations in the anatomic or physiologic condition of the vocal tract, clients may outgrow them or the problems may continue past the developmental period and require treatment.

diadochokinetic tasks   Tasks used to evaluate the maximum repetition rate of different articulators. The repetitive stimuli generally consist of syllables and provide an index of speech motor control.

diphthongs   Sounds produced with an open vocal tract and made by changing from one vowel articulation to another in the same syllable nuclei (see also *vowels*).

distortion errors   Variants of intended target sounds that are nonallophonic and not other phonemes.

drill   Therapeutic treatment procedure that is highly structured and designed to elicit multiple practice responses from the client.

drill/play   Therapeutic treatment procedure that is similar to drill but differs in terms of the use of some motivational activity such as a game to elicit practice responses.

durational information   Information regarding various aspects of speech timing such as vowel length. This type of data furnishes cues that speakers may use in speech perception.

dynamic range   Difference in decibels between a client's hearing threshold of sensitivity for sound and the level at which sound is uncomfortably loud.

dysarthria   Motor speech disorder exhibiting difficulty with the execution of articulatory movements and possibly other components of speech production such as respiration, phonation, resonation, and prosody as the result of central or peripheral nervous system damage.

dyskinetic dysarthria   Motor speech disorder that is the result of injury to the basal ganglia, a group of nuclei located at the base of the cerebral hemispheres. The major perceptual speech features are articulatory imprecision and voice problems.

electropalatography   Instrumentation that detects tongue-palate contacts during speech via the placement of an artificial palate. A physiologic biofeedback signal is provided for the learner.

expiratory function   Measurement or estimation of subglottal pressure for speech through either speech or nonspeech tasks.

expressive representations   Component of a theory proposed by Straight (1980)* (see also *receptive representations*).

feature contrasts   Category of phonological process errors such as the stopping of fricatives that consist of substitutions of place or manner features (or substitutions of both).

feedback   Motor learning concept regarding the analysis of performance information by the learner. This type of information is internalized from practice trials through various forms of sensory information and conscious introspection.

flaccid dysarthria   Motor speech disorder that is the result of injury to the lower motor neurons located in the brainstem and spinal cord that innervate the speech musculature, the cranial and spinal nerves, or the actual muscle fibers that the nerves innervate. The major perceptual speech features are weak articulatory contacts, breathy voice quality, and hypernasality.

formants   Resonances or peaks in the amplitude spectrum of the vocal tract during speech production. Formants vary as a function of changes in the configuration of the vocal tract.

frequency   Number of cycles of vibration of a sound-producing mechanism such as the vocal folds. Its measurement is carried out in hertz (Hz).

fricatives   Class of consonant speech sounds produced by forcing air, acoustic sound energy, or both through a narrow vocal tract constriction. The speech sounds in this class are /f, v, θ, ð, s, z, ʃ, h, ʒ/.

glides   Speech sounds produced by shifting or gliding from one position to another position in the same syllable. Glides are also classified as *oral semivowels*. The glide speech sounds are /w, j/.

---

*Straight HSS: Auditory versus articulatory processes and their development in children. In Yeni-Komshian GH, Kavanagh JF, Ferguson CA, editors: *Child Phonology Volume 1: production*, New York, 1980, Academic Press.

glottal stop Stop sound produced by complete occlusion of the vocal folds followed by a quick release. Some speakers with cleft palate use the substitution as a compensatory articulation. Glottal stop is an allophonic variant of /t/ or /d/ for some normal speakers.

groping Oral silent posturing of articulatory positions before production. Groping is sometimes reported as a symptom associated with childhood apraxia of speech (CAS).

hard-of-hearing Term used to describe clients classified as having a *mild, moderate,* or *severe hearing loss.*

harmony (assimilation) Phonological process error that reflects context-sensitive sound change. One of the contrasting target consonants in a word assumes the features of another consonant in that word.

homonymy Collapse of phonemic contrast or contrasts so that the client produces one sound in substitution of a single or several adult sounds.

hypernasality Perception of nasal resonance during the production of voiced sounds, particularly vowels.

hypoglossia Abnormally small tongue.

hypoglossia-hypodactyly sequence Relatively rare birth anomaly with major features consisting of a partial to total absence of the tongue and of the digits of one or more limbs.

"inspiratory checking" Technique designed to improve the coordination of breathing during speech production. The client is instructed to inhale deeply and then exhale slowly when producing speech.

intelligibility drills Therapy treatment procedure that uses minimal-pair word sets that the client produces and the clinician identifies.

interdental fricatives Fricative sounds made with the tongue slightly protruded between the upper and lower incisors (see also *fricatives*). These include /θ, ð/.

internal phonological knowledge Person's internal knowledge of the ways that sound categories are used to signal meaning differences and permissible ways that the sound categories are used in morpheme construction.

knowledge of results (KR) Motor learning concept that pertains to performance information provided to the client by an external source such as the clinician. KR can be qualitative, quantitative, or both.

labiodental fricatives Fricative sounds made with the upper incisors and lower lip (see also *fricatives*). These are /f, v/.

liquids Sounds produced with a relatively open vocal tact, similar to that of vowels, and also classified as *oral semivowels.* They are /r, l/.

macroglossia Enlarged tongue.

major class differences Primary class features that differentiate among classes of speech sounds. These include vowels versus consonants, consonants versus glides, and sonorants versus obstruents.

markedness Construct pertaining to the linguistic properties of languages. This preferred feature in a language implies an unmarked feature. For example, voicing is an example of this type of feature and implies an opposite feature of voicelessness. Phonological treatment approaches use this construct in the selection of treatment targets. Accordingly, the clinician should teach the preferred feature to facilitate the acquisition of its opposite.

maximal opposition Contrastive approach to phonological therapy that pairs a sound that is missing from the client's inventory with a sound that is functional in the child's inventory, or one that pairs sounds that are both missing from the child's inventory. In either case the contrastive pairs are selected to reflect major or nonmajor feature differences.

metaphon approach   Treatment that targets phonological processes primarily through the use of metalinguistic awareness tasks with minimal attention to the production of phonemic contrasts.

middorsum palatal stop   Compensatory articulation used in substitution for /t/, /d/, /k/, or /g/ by some children with velopharyngeal dysfunction, palatal fistulae, or both.

minimal pairs   Phonological treatment approach that contrasts the child's error with the target sound in an effort to eliminate homonymy.

mixed dysarthria   Motor speech disorder with speech symptoms that reflect diffuse damage of the motor system.

mixed hearing loss   Hearing loss with both conductive and sensorineural components. Management of this type of loss will depend on the contributions of each component.

motor skill learning   Type of learning consisting of principles developed to teach simple and complex motor skills. The principles and underlying theory have been adapted to teaching children and adults with sound system disorders.

motor speech disorders   Neurologically based speech disorders that may exhibit problems with motor planning, coordination of muscle movement, timing of movements, or implementation of the movement patterns requisite to normal speech production (or a combination of these problems). In addition to an articulatory component, these disorders may also include involvement of other biocommunication systems such as respiration, phonation, resonation, and speech prosody.

multiple oppositions   Phonological treatment that targets multiple phoneme collapse through the use of contrast. Several target sounds are contrasted with a comparison sound simultaneously.

multiple phoneme collapse   Collapse of a phonemic contrast that is present in the adult system. It may be across several adult sounds so that the child uses a single sound to represent several different adult sounds.

nasal emission   Presence of air escaping through the nose during the production of pressure sounds, particularly voiceless pressure sounds. It may be audible or inaudible.

nasal murmur   Acoustic phenomenon that reflects a production feature of nasal sounds. It manifests as a major low-frequency resonance or nasal formant.

nasal snort   Compensatory articulation produced by channeling air directly through the nasal tract. The production is used frequently in place of fricatives and also referred to as a *posterior nasal fricative*.

nasal turbulence   Form of nasal emission. Air passes through the nasal cavity and may set tissue into vibration, or air is forced into a narrowed constriction, possibly because of a nasal obstruction. Nasal turbulence is perceived as a nasal rustle or turbulent noise.

National Outcome Measurement System (NOMS)   Project that is being conducted by the American Speech-Language-Hearing Association (ASHA) for the purpose of collecting outcome data on the treatment of speech, swallowing, and language disorders.

naturalistic play   Collection of different play activities used to elicit desired target responses. The clinician may use different elicitation techniques such as self-talk and modeling to promote the production of target responses.

naturalness   Perceptual term used to describe the adequacy or inadequacy of prosody for a particular speaker.

neighborhood density   Metric of the number of words that differ minimally in phonetic makeup from a specific word in terms of a single phoneme substitution, deletion, or addition.

nonce item   Sound combination that is not a morpheme and may or may not have a permissible phonological structure. A nonce item is generally paired with a picture or line drawing (to associate meaning with the nonce item) and is used to reduce phoneme interference.

nonmajor class features   Features of voice, place, and manner used to delineate the production attributes of individual sounds. For example, /p/ is a voiceless bilabial stop. These features differ from their counterpart, major differences, which distinguish among the primary categories of sound production such as vowels versus consonants.

obligatory errors   Function of structural problems that have adverse effects on the physiologic movement or movements requisite to correct sound production. They are generally not subject to speech treatment and are sometimes referred to as *passive speech characteristics*.

open bite   Presence of a gap or opening between the anterior maxillary and mandibular teeth.

operant learning   Theory of learning that uses the instructional cycle of stimulus-response-reinforcement when teaching various behaviors such as sound system production.

Opitz syndrome   Syndrome that may include craniofacial, genitourinary, gastrointestinal, central nervous system, and cardiac involvement. Speech and language skills are generally delayed, with possible neurologic association. Compensatory errors may be present if a cleft of the palate exists.

oral-facial-digital syndrome   Group of eight different disorder types that are genetically different but grouped together because of similar phenotype expression. Major clinical features may include craniofacial, limbs, skin, central nervous system, and kidney problems. Speech disorders may be the result of abnormal tongue anatomy and enlarged oral frenulae.

oral-facial-digital syndrome, type I   See *oral-facial-digital syndrome.*

oral motor treatment (OMT)   Collection of treatments that target nonspeech oral motor movements and oral postures with the aim of developing motor patterns requisite for speech sound production, strengthening the muscles used in speech production, or both.

oronasal fistulae   Breakdowns in tissue at the site of surgical closure of the palate that result in an opening into the nasal passages.

otitis media   Inflammation of the middle ear that may exhibit no obvious symptoms.

palatal fricatives   Fricative sounds made at the palatal point of articulation. They are /ʃ, ʒ/ (see also *fricatives*).

palatal lift   Prosthetic speech appliance used to improve velopharyngeal closure for speech, generally in cases of neurologic impairment to the velum.

passive speech characteristics   Speech disorders that are the result of a structural problem such as a velopharyngeal closure deficit. Problems such as hypernasality, nasal emission, and weak pressure consonant production are examples. These are also referred to as *obligatory errors.*

pharyngeal fricative   Compensatory error produced by creating a narrow constriction with the tongue base and pharyngeal wall and then channeling air through the constriction.

pharyngeal stop   Compensatory error produced via tongue dorsum and pharyngeal wall occlusion and quick release.

pharyngoplasty   Surgical procedure of the pharynx used to correct velopharyngeal dysfunction.

phoneme contrast   Aim of phonological treatment—to create phonemic distinctions that are nonexistent in a client's system. Minimal pairs, multiple oppositions, and maximal oppositions are examples of contrastive treatments.

phoneme-specific nasal emission   Emission of air through the nose during the production of one or more pressure sounds. The cause is mislearning rather than structurally or neurologically based, and the problem is amenable to speech treatment.

phonemic   Adjective that refers to phonemes (the sounds of the language) that contrast and signal semantic distinctiveness.

phonetic   Adjective that pertains to the perceptual, physiologic, or acoustic properties of the sounds of a language.

phonetic placement   Instructional technique for teaching sound placement. The clinician uses verbal instructions and diagrams regarding placement of the articulators in sound elicitation trials.

phonological knowledge   Person's knowledge of the sound system of a language. Phonological knowledge is a composite of acoustic-perceptual knowledge, articulatory-phonetic knowledge, and internal knowledge.

phonotactic constraints   Phonological rules that restrict the incidence of particular sounds or sound sequences from a client's phonetic and phonemic inventories. These include inventory constraints, positional constraints, and sequence constraints.

physiologic biofeedback   Provision of feedback to the learner in the form of some physiologic signal that is typically not available on a conscious level. Aerodynamic, electromyographic, and electropalatographic information are examples of signals used in this type of feedback.

plosive cognates   See *cognates.*

plosives   See *stops.*

primary reinforcers   Consequents directed to the biologic or physiologic needs (or both) of the client. Desirable foods are sometimes used to reinforce wanted behaviors.

prosodic features   See *prosody.*

prosody   Suprasegmental speech features superimposed on phonetic units such as syllables, words, phrases, and sentences. Some of these features include stress, intonation, loudness, pitch level, juncture, and speaking rate.

prosthesis   Intraoral device fabricated by a prosthodontist for the purpose of improving speech production, swallowing, or both. Some clients are fitted with this device to improve velopharyngeal closure for speech.

prosthetic placement cues   Type of oral appliance used outside or inside the oral cavity for the purpose of positioning the articulators to elicit a specific target sound.

prosthodontist   Dental specialist who fabricates speech prostheses.

random sequencing   Motor learning concept wherein all levels of a treatment are administered randomly to the client within a single treatment session. It generally results in reduced response accuracy rates per session but greater generalization when compared with block sequencing.

rapport   Development of a supportive relationship between the practitioner and client and between the practitioner and parent.

recasts   Form of naturalistic conversation-based teaching. The clinician points out the client's errors during conversational interchanges designed to create client awareness of target errors while not detracting from the "naturalness" of the conversational interchange.

receptive representations   Component of a theory proposed by Straight (1980) in which a speaker of the language has the underlying representations of individual morphemes stored internally. The underlying representations are abstract accounts that include a semantic component and the learned phonological characteristics of the morpheme. The *receptive* forms include the auditory features of words that the child can understand, whereas the *expressive* forms contain the articulatory features of the words that the child can produce.

reduced intraoral pressure   Plosive, fricative, and affricate sounds are produced with insufficient air buildup because of velopharyngeal dysfunction, palatal fistulae, or both.

residual errors   Subtype of sound system errors. These do not normalize through maturation, or in some cases after treatment, and continue past the expected period of speech sound acquisition for some clients.

response generalization   Generalization of target behaviors to behaviors that have not been taught to the client.

secondary reinforcers   Reinforcers that are of intrinsic value to the learner. Forms such as verbal praise, token economies, and performance feedback are used frequently in treatments using operant learning.

See-Scape   Inexpensive low-technology instrument that detects the presence of nasal emission.

segmental errors   Sound errors present in a client's speech.

semivowels   Sounds made with a relatively open vocal tract to allow for cavity resonance. The semivowels are /j/, /w/, /l/, /r/, /m/, /n/, and /ŋ/.

sensorineural hearing loss   Type of hearing loss that is the result of damage to the sensory end organ of hearing, damage to the cochlear hair cells, or a pathologic condition of the auditory nerve.

slit fricatives   Fricative sounds made with an elliptic rather than circular orifice. These include /f/, /v/, /θ/, and /ð/.

sonorant feature   Sound made with a relatively unconstricted vocal tract. Liquids, nasals, vowels, and glides share this feature.

sound pressure   Sound intensity measured in terms of sound pressure level, which is the amount of force per unit area.

sound spectrograph   Instrument that allows the acoustic analysis of sound via a visual display of frequency, intensity, and duration parameters.

spastic dysarthria   Motor speech disorder caused by damage to the upper motor neuron system. The upper motor neuron system includes cortical motor areas and associative areas that are direct or indirect pathways for connection with lower motor neurons located in the brainstem and spinal cord. The major perceptual speech features are vocal harshness, hypernasality, imprecise consonants, and reduced speaking rate.

spectral information   Data composed of frequency and intensity variations of the speech signal that are available to listeners for the perception of speech.

speech appliances   Prosthetic intraoral devices used for some clients with velopharyngeal closure deficits or palatal fistulae. They can be used in cases of tissue deficiency or lack of velar movement.

speech intelligibility   Index used to estimate the speech that can be understood by a hearing-impaired listener (when taken in the context of hearing impairment). Intelligibility is a complex function of frequency, intensity, and duration. In the context of a client who has a sound system disorder without hearing impairment, this is the comprehensibility of the client's spontaneous speech by a listener.

speech intensity   Sound energy of the speech signal that is measured in decibels. The perceptual correlate of intensity is loudness.

speed drill   Therapy technique used in phonetic teaching that is used to automate target sounds via timed drills.

stimulus generalization   Learned response to a specific stimulus that is evoked by comparable stimuli.

stop sounds   Class of consonant speech sounds that require a complete closure of the vocal tract followed by a quick release of air, acoustic sound energy, or both. They are /p, b, t, d, k, g/.

structural defects   Anatomic anomalies of the vocal tract that may be minor in nature, such as missing teeth, or major, such as cleft lip and palate. These may or may not adversely affect speech production skills.

structured play   Treatment activities that are presented in play-type activities, particularly in cases in which the child does not respond to more formal modes of instruction.

substitution errors   Errors in which one sound is substituted in place of another sound and generally reflects changes in the place or manner of articulation (or changes in both).

suprasegmentals   See *prosody.*

syllable structure   Unit of speech with a nucleus that is generally a vowel. The vowel may be preceded or followed by (or preceded and followed by) single- or multiple-consonant segments.

tense/lax pairs   Contrastive terms that refer to the production feature of muscular tension in vowels. The first describes vowels produced with greater lingual tension that also are longer in duration than the latter type.

tongue blade   Wooden blade used to position and observe the oral articulators.

training trial   Therapy event that culminates in a client response. Response accuracy data are collected for the client's performance across individual events.

ultrasound   Imaging medium that uses high-frequency sound waves to identify the anatomy of interest.

velar fricative   Compensatory sound substitution produced at a constriction point of the tongue dorsum and velum.

velars Sounds made at the velar point of articulation, such as the plosives /k/ and /g/.

velopharyngeal dysfunction Lack of complete closure of the velopharyngeal mechanism during speech, which generally results in the presence of hypernasality, nasal emission, and possibly compensatory errors.

vocalic transitions Changes in the formant frequencies of a vowel as the result of sounds that precede and follow it. These provide important speech perception information to listeners.

voice onset time (VOT) Interval between the release of an oral consonant and the start of laryngeal vibration for the following vowel. This is an important variable in the production of prevocalic stops.

vowels Class of speech sounds produced with sound energy created by vocal fold vibration, which resonates through a relatively open vocal tract of a particular configuration. Vowel production is primarily a function of the movement of the lips, tongue, and jaw.

water manometer Glass tube filled with liquid that is used to measure air pressure.

wooden dowel Small wooden shaft inserted between the molar teeth that is used to stabilize the jaw for sound elicitation.

word frequency Regularity at which a particular word occurs in a language.

X-linked cleft palate Birth defect that is inherited in a sex-linked manner and sometimes found in combination with ankyloglossia.

Index

Page numbers followed by *b* indicate boxes;
f, figures; *t*, tables.